THE SCIENCE OF BECOMING

A medical approach to self-transformation

DR J CRESPO

Rethink

First published in Great Britain in 2026
by Rethink Press (www.rethinkpress.com)

Cover artwork by Cuttlefish Studio, cuttlefishstudio.co.uk

Disclaimer: Though I am a doctor, this book is not intended as medical advice. It is meant as an aid for those that would like to become an improved version of themselves, using published medical principles and evidence as well as life experiences. All the patients' examples included in this book are used to illustrate real concepts and experiences and they have been altered to make identification impossible, even by the patients themselves.

Contents

Introduction 1

The doctor who chose to heal 4

1 Identifying Who You Are 7

The medical foundation of identity 8

Beyond personality tests – biological variables that shape identity 11

The neuroplasticity revolution 15

The integration challenge 17

Practical identity discovery 19

Take-home messages 22

2 Identifying Your Goals 25

The neuroscience of goal setting 27

HEAL goals: A sound approach 30

The biological reality of motivation 32

Goal hierarchy: Foundations first 37

The energy equation 39

The authenticity filter 43

Practical goal design 45

The compound effect of aligned goals 47
Emotional harmony – the musical analogy 49
Take-home messages 50

3 Identifying Your Health: The Physical, Foundation-Creating Health 53

The prevention revolution 55
The inflammation epidemic 59
Foundation health markers 65
The movement medicine 67
Sleep: The ultimate performance enhancer 72
The nutrition foundation 75
Recovery: The missing piece 76
The physical integration blueprint 77
Take-home messages 79

4 Identifying Your Stress: Mental And Emotional Wellness 81

The system that connects body, mind and emotion 82
The stress response revolution 86
The trauma factor that most ignore 90
The science of emotional control 91
The gut–brain revolution 98
Practical mental and emotional wellness 101
Take-home messages 104

5 Longevity: Living Better, Not Just Longer 107

Redefining success in personal development 107

The longevity diet paradox 110
The science of ageing: From inevitable to modifiable 111
Evidence-based longevity interventions 118
Decoding the biohacking movement: Where science ends and marketing begins 121
The blue zones solution: Secrets of the world's healthiest people 123
Longevity and personal transformation 124
Take-home messages 127

6 Identifying Your Optimal Nutrition: Science Or Sensationalism? 131
The nutrition information paradox 132
The foundation: Understanding your biochemistry 135
The science of fasting 140
Finding your individual 146
Take-home messages 150

7 Relationships: The Social Prescription 153
The medical case for relationships 156
Family relationships: The first blueprint 159
The friendship prescription 160
Marriage and partnership: The health benefits 161
Loneliness 163
The social skills that build connection 166
The ripple effect of relationships 168

Take-home messages 169

8 Love: The Neuroscience Of Connection 171

Love is medicine 172

The architecture of love 178

Love: The bridge to becoming 181

Take-home messages 182

9 Creating The New You: Evidence-Based Transformation 185

Integration: A whole-person approach 186

The neuroscience of change 187

The power of silence: Meditation science 193

Beyond meditation: Other transformative practices 196

The change process: A medical model 197

Becoming who you truly are 204

Take-home messages 205

Conclusion: Your Journey Begins Now 207

References 211

Further Reading 233

Acknowledgements 241

The Author 245

Introduction

You've tried everything. The morning rituals, the meditation apps, the life coaches, the self-help books that pledged transformation in thirty days or your money back. You may even have succeeded by external measures – a brilliant career, a comfortable home, respectable relationships. Despite all your achievements, though, something inside feels missing. Not sadness exactly and not quite depression. Just a persistent sense of not being fully alive.

Maybe you climbed the ladder only to discover that it was leaning on the wrong wall. Perhaps you are the parent giving everything to everyone else while slowly fading in the background. Or maybe you've applied all the recommended habits and mindset shifts but still find yourself repeating the same frustrating patterns.

If any of this resonates, you may feel broken, but let me be clear: you are not. Your struggle isn't due to a lack of willpower or motivation. It stems from a disconnect between the desire to change and your understanding of how change actually happens.

Many people assume this struggle is purely psychological, but the truth is more profound: your biology and your psychology are inseparable. The chemistry of your brain, the balance of your hormones, the sensitivity of your nervous system, the inflammatory load of your gut microbiome – all are shaping your thoughts, emotions and behaviours every single day.

You cannot think your way out of a problem that has deep biological roots. Psychological strategies can certainly help, but they're simply more effective when the underlying biology is also supported.

Traditional self-help approaches often conceptualise people like malfunctioning machines – just upgrade your mindset, improve your discipline or reconfigure your habits, and everything will fall into place. These approaches address isolated symptoms rather than addressing the whole human system. Affirmations alone will not balance cortisol. Motivation alone cannot override a malfunctioning thyroid. Positive thinking alone will not stabilise sugar levels.

The science of becoming is not about forcing yourself into a new identity. It's about understanding the biology that makes identity, behaviour and emotions possible in the first place. Transformation is not an act of force; it is a process of alignment.

In the chapters ahead you will not find promises of instant transformation. Real change, like the healing of a broken bone, follows biological processes and can't be rushed. It requires time, coherence and proper conditions.

What you'll learn is how biology and psychology work together, how to overcome hurdles to sustain change and how to build a system in which growth is the natural outcome rather than a daily battle. *The Science of Becoming* uses medical evidence to make meaningful personal change accessible and biologically grounded.

Your biology is not your enemy. When understood and supported, it will become your greatest ally.

Your becoming is deeply personal at first, of course, but it never stops there. When you become true to yourself, you encourage others to do the same. When you start living from a place of aligned purpose, you generate ripples of positive influence that spread outward and benefit more than just your own life. This is the potential of real transformation – it begins with you, but it doesn't end with you, and you don't have to walk it by yourself.

The doctor who chose to heal

I was not always a doctor. For years I wore expensive suits instead of scrubs and checked spreadsheets instead of X-rays. I supposedly had it all – the office overlooking London, business class flights around the world, a good salary. Here's the thing about success, though: it can become a beautiful prison. I had everything I thought I wanted yet somehow felt adrift. Every morning I'd wake up with a hollow sense that I was living someone else's life. Only then did I stop running from the voice that had been whispering to me since childhood, which I had drowned out with practical life decisions and other people's expectations. This was my calling *to become.*

I'd learned a lot in the corporate world. As a lawyer I realised the real story always lies beneath what people tell you and that you have to probe further, asking the uncomfortable questions. In finance I learned the difference between a quick profit and building something that lasts. Both careers gave me a bird's-eye view of problems and the ability to identify patterns others missed.

Little did I know, these skills would later be my secret weapons in medicine. Walking into medical school felt surreal. There I was, with students in their twenties who absorbed anatomy like sponges, while I was still figuring out where to sit. I brought something they didn't, though: battle scars. I'd seen successful people collapse behind closed doors and watched brilliant minds destroy themselves with alcohol and pills, all while maintaining perfect facades because admitting struggle felt like failure.

I purposely didn't follow the traditional path through prestigious teaching hospitals. Instead, I chose to work in understaffed district hospitals; and in maximum security prisons, where I met hardened criminals who broke down sobbing the moment someone listened to their stories. I watched healing occur in dusty medical camps across India, with nothing but human touch and hope. No fancy equipment, no miracle drugs – just presence. That's when it all hit me: suffering and the ability to heal aren't correlated with postcodes. I have dealt with foreign royalty and millionaire executives with access to the world's best specialists who were consumed by anxiety and despair. The same principles that change lives in prison cells are true in penthouses. Our medical system is amazing at fixing what's broken but lousy at keeping people whole. We can repair hearts, but we can't stop people from eating foods that destroy them. We have treatments that save lives but struggle to address the loneliness that's killing us from the inside out, and many people, regardless of culture or social status, feel they are struggling to cope with daily life challenges.

Here's what I need you to understand: you're not broken. You don't need fixing. Everything you need for inner change already exists within you; we just need to create the right conditions for it to flourish. Your transformation starts with you, but it never ends there.

Transformation begins long before action. It begins with understanding the version of yourself you have been unconsciously living, which is shaped by biology, history and survival strategies you never chose. When you finally see the architecture of your identity, the possibility of becoming someone new – someone authentic – emerges.

Let's begin.

ONE
Identifying Who You Are

Sarah, a forty-two-year-old marketing executive, sat across from me, exhausted but composed. On paper she had everything she'd ever thought she wanted: a large office, a six-figure salary, a beautiful house, a full social life and widespread praise for her work excellence. However, internally she felt detached, as if she was living someone else's life.

'Doctor,' she whispered, 'I don't even recognise who I am anymore.'

Sarah's question, one I often hear in my clinic, made me reflect on how we have been taught to approach identity and growth. For decades books like *The 7 Habits of Highly Effective People* (Covey, 1989) have suggested that identity is built through roles and objectives.

Although there is great merit in this approach, it overlooks a foundational truth: identity does not begin with behaviour; it begins with biology.

Who you are – including your preferences, tendencies, fears and motivations – is shaped by millions of biological signals travelling through your body: hormones, neurotransmitters, immune activity, sensory input, memories, emotional imprints, gut bacteria and nervous systems patterns laid down across decades. These signals form the *felt sense* of you.

When those biological signals are balanced, the self feels coherent. When they are dysregulated, the self feels fragmented. It is very difficult to know who you truly are when your biology is working against you.

When I identified Sarah's thyroid imbalance and chronic low-grade inflammation, her sense of self shifted. Her energy returned to undertake activities she had abandoned, her thinking sharpened, and her mood stabilised. She felt, in her words, 'like myself again'. This was not a personality change. It was the removal of biological interference that had been masking her true personality.

The medical foundation of identity

Modern neuroscience demonstrates that there is no line separating mind and body. The brain and the body are in constant dialogue.

Antonio Damasio's research (1994, 2010) provides evidence against the traditional idea of mind: Body duality. In *Descartes' Error* he introduces the 'somatic marker hypothesis', suggesting that bodily signals such as changes in heart rate, gut sensation and hormonal shifts play a critical role in guiding reasoning and decision-making processes. In *Self Comes to* Mind, he further explains how the sense of the self is not independent from the body but emerges from the continuous mapping of internal bodily states in the brain. The neural systems responsible for emotion and decision-making are closely integrated with the regions that monitor the body's internal environment. This helps explain why some people may do extensive psychological work yet still find change difficult – not because the psychological work is ineffective but because biological and emotional systems also need to be supported. Without addressing the physiological signals that shape emotion and sense of self, the picture remains incomplete.

Dr Candace Pert expanded our scientific understanding of emotions through her breakthrough discovery of the brain's opioid receptor. Her research revealed that the emotion signalling system of neuropeptides extends throughout the entire body, with receptors present not only in the brain but also distributed across the body's cells (Pert et al, 1985). These networks of receptors receive the chemical messages that encode emotional states such as joy, fear and sadness (Pert, 1997).

Even more surprisingly, Pert found that the entire lining of the intestine is populated with neuropeptide receptors, explaining why so often we feel emotions in our gut. As she concluded in *Molecules of Emotion* (Pert, 1997), 'the body is the unconscious mind'. Pert's work illuminated the profound biochemical dialogue between mind and body, but this should not be confused with modern claims about peptide supplementation. Her research does not validate commercial peptide products.

Your body does not simply respond to your emotions. It participates in creating them. A tightened chest, a surge of warmth, a heavy stomach, a sense of joy – these are not mere reactions to thoughts but biological signals informing the brain of meaning – threat, safety or opportunity. Identity is therefore not purely a psychological phenomenon. It is an embodied pattern – a biological signature. When your biology is imbalanced, through inflammation, hormone disruption, nutrient deficiencies or chronic stress, your sense of self can become distorted.

Biology is frequently oversimplified, and Pert's discoveries inadvertently contributed to the modern fascination with peptide-based therapies. Today synthetic peptides are promoted widely. Some are well researched, medically supervised and, in the right context, they can play a legitimate therapeutic role. With their enthusiasm for these synthetic peptides, though, people often misinterpret the science.

The peptides Pert studied were not isolated chemicals acting independently. They were part of the body's refined, evolution-shaped signalling network: neuropeptides coordinating communication between the brain, gut and immune system to shape emotion, behaviour and the felt sense of self.

Unsupervised use of synthetic peptides risks disturbing a delicate signalling network whose full dynamics we still do not understand. Modern neuroscience – from Damasio's somatic marker hypothesis to Pert's work on neuropeptides – confirms that every thought and feeling is rooted in physical processes. Any intervention that interferes with those processes requires caution, precision and scientific humility.

In short: peptides can be therapeutic, but they are not shortcuts to self-reinvention.

Beyond personality tests: Biological variables that shape identity

Personality tests such as Myers-Briggs (1995), Enneagram (Riso and Hudson, 1999) and StrengthsFinder (Gallup and Rath, 2007) are widely used in workplaces and personal development settings. Some of my patients have tried them, hoping to better understand themselves. These tests can provide helpful insights, but they overlook one very important thing: your biology.

Four biological variables can influence how you experience yourself on a daily basis:

1. **Chronotype:** Your natural rhythm
2. **Stress-response pattern:** How your cortisol rises and falls
3. **Neurotransmitter profile:** The balance of chemicals such as dopamine and serotonin
4. **Inflammatory baseline:** The silent biological driver of mood and energy

1. Chronotype

Do you work better early in the morning or late in the evening? This is not a matter of laziness or preference; it is largely dictated by your genes, and it influences your mood, thinking patterns and emotional stability. Your chronotype determines when your brain is at its sharpest, when you are most creative and even the best time for you to have a stressful conversation. According to chronobiological research, chronotype affects far more than just when you sleep; it also influences mood, stress levels, cognitive performance, decision-making and overall health across the day (Roenneberg et al, 2012).

Sonia, a thirty-year-old marketing executive, spent years participating in early-morning meetings when her body was still in melatonin-dominant 'night mode'. When she rearranged her schedule to align with her natural rhythm, her productivity increased and her anxiety decreased significantly.

2. Stress-response pattern

Some people naturally produce higher levels of cortisol, which helps them function well in a crisis but makes it harder for them to relax. Others have a more muted stress response, allowing them to remain calm under pressure, but this can make them appear less driven. Sapolsky's research (Sapolsky, 2004) shows that such patterns are shaped by both genetics and early life experiences, creating unique *stress signatures* that influence our career preferences, relationships and daily behaviour.

Understanding your stress-response pattern allows you to structure life in a way that supports your nervous system. If you have a high-activation stress response, you thrive with regular, intense physical activity and planned periods of rest. If you have a more muted response, novelty, stimulation and varied environments help keep you engaged and motivated.

3. Neurotransmitter profile

Dopamine, serotonin, norepinephrine and other neurotransmitters influence motivation, sociability, focus and sensitivity. You may be naturally optimistic or cautious, social or solitary, detail-orientated or big-picture-focused, depending in part on your baseline levels of these neurotransmitters. Neurotransmitter functioning can be influenced by lifestyle choices, but understanding your baseline can help you make decisions that feel more satisfying and sustainable.

The brain's neurotransmitter system is complex, and research into how it may shape personality is ongoing.

4. Inflammatory baseline

Some people have genetic variants that predispose them to higher levels of inflammation, which can affect mood, energy and cognitive function, which are sometimes wrongly attributed to personality.

Research from Pariante (2017) shows that chronic low-grade inflammation can produce symptoms almost identical to depression, anxiety and attention disorders.

Michael, a software engineer, came to me believing he was lazy and demotivated. The self-help books he'd read over the years had simply reinforced what he perceived as personal failings. When we tested his genetics, we found variants affecting his dopamine metabolism and vitamin D absorption. With targeted supplementation, adjusted sun exposure, and training based on his genetic profile, his 'personality' shifted. He was no longer the lazy person he thought he was.

While these biological variables influence personality, research in this area is still evolving. Current evidence shows correlations rather than fixed or deterministic personality patterns.

Personality is not fixed. It is shaped by the constant interaction between your genes and your environment. When you understand and optimise your biology, you often unlock abilities you never realised you had.

Biology shapes identity, but biology is also changeable.

The neuroplasticity revolution

The point that most self-help teachers get right though often oversimplify is that your brain can reorganise itself throughout life – a phenomenon known as *neuroplasticity*. This means that the pathways shaping your habits, reactions and sense of self are not fixed. Research by Doidge (2007) has shown that the neural pathways underlying your behaviour and identity remain malleable and that the patterns in your mind are changeable. In other words, you can rewire your brain to support you in becoming your authentic self.

However, neuroplasticity is biologically dependent. Your brain remodels itself more effectively when certain foundations are in place:

- High-quality sleep
- Stable blood glucose
- Emotional safety

- Adequate nutrition
- Low inflammation

The work of Merzenich (2013) demonstrates that neuroplasticity operates through specific principles:

1. **Focus:** Neuroplastic change accelerates when you engage in intense, concentrated practice on a new skill or behaviour. Distracted practice reinforces existing patterns rather than building new ones.
2. **Progressive challenge:** Effective learning occurs when tasks gradually increase in difficulty, becoming challenging enough to require effort (what researchers call *optimal challenge*) but achievable enough to maintain motivation and avoid frustration.
3. **Repetition and consistency:** Neural networks strengthen through repeated activation. Sporadic practice, regardless of intensity, cannot establish lasting neural pathways.
4. **Emotional relevance:** Changes that resonate with your values and emotions become more deeply encoded in the brain than any purely intellectual changes.
5. **Consolidation and recovery:** Sleep and downtime allow your brain to consolidate new neural connections. Sustainable meaningful change requires recovery, not effort alone.

Many people attempt to change their behaviour while their physiology is unstable, and this makes progress far more difficult. Biology always sets the boundaries of transformation.

Maria, a fifty-five-year-old teacher, had always assumed she was naturally anxious and pessimistic. Once she corrected a magnesium deficiency, treated her sleep apnoea and stabilised the hormonal distress of perimenopause, she discovered wells of calm and optimism she previously hadn't thought possible. Her personality was never the problem; her biological dysfunction was.

Remember that identity is not created. It is revealed when biology and environment stop competing with each other.

The integration challenge

Books such as *Atomic Habits* (Clear, 2018) rightly emphasise that lasting change arises not from altering your behaviours but from shifting the underlying identity. *Your self-image is important.* If you see yourself as someone who exercises regularly, maintaining that behaviour becomes far easier than if your aim is, for example, simply to exercise for weight loss.

Where this popular approach falls short is in the assumption that we can simply choose a new identity and that willpower alone is all it takes. I have learned that transformation lives or dies in the space between your biology and your intentions. No amount of willpower can override biology that is signalling resistance – physiology sets the conditions in which new identities can take hold.

When I help patients explore identity and self-concept, I often suggest undertaking a comprehensive wellness review:

1. **Hormone levels:** Energy, drive and emotional stability are all influenced by testosterone, oestrogen, thyroid hormones and cortisol. Low testosterone (in both men and women) can reduce drive and ambition. Thyroid dysfunction can mimic apathy and low mood. Chronic stress dysregulates cortisol, impairing decision-making and persistence.

2. **Nutrient status:** Deficiencies in B vitamins, omega-3 fatty acids, magnesium and vitamin D alter mood, cognition and emotional regulation. These nutrients are cofactors in neurotransmitter production and neuroplasticity. When they are suboptimal, identity change is biologically resisted because the brain lacks the resources to support new patterns.

3. **Inflammatory markers:** Low-grade chronic inflammation clouds the brain and flattens mood. Elevated inflammatory markers such as C-reactive protein and homocysteine can

contribute to brain fog and reduced self-awareness, making reflection and behavioural change far more difficult.

4. **Sleep quality:** Sleep deprivation undermines emotional regulation and impairs the prefrontal cortex, the region of the brain responsible for self-control, planning and perspective. Without adequate sleep, no identity shift can stabilise.
5. **Gut health:** Your microbiome communicates with your brain via the gut–brain axis. If your microbiome is not balanced, it can create anxiety, depressive symptoms and cognitive dysfunction.

Practical identity discovery

My patients have taught me that genuine self-discovery tends to follow a predictable pattern. The approach I use is:

- Step 1: Optimise your biology before identity work
- Step 2: Observe without judgement
- Step 3: Respect your natural rhythms
- Step 4: Experiment with enhancement

Step 1: Optimise your biology before identity work

First and foremost, it is always best to address your physical health before diving into psychological and emotional identity work. You cannot discover the real you when your body is working against you. Addressing your physical health includes getting enough sleep, stabilising blood glucose, balancing hormones and reducing inflammation. Before exploring your true identity, tune it. Like instruments before a concert, begin by calibrating the biology you were born with.

In practice, it is often necessary first to build trust by listening to a patient's emotional or mood-expressive concerns, before guiding them towards the physical assessment that will support deeper identity work.

Step 2: Observe without judgement

This observational period is an essential next step. For one or two weeks it is necessary to keep a simple log of:

- Energy levels throughout the day
- Mood fluctuations and their triggers
- Activities that uplift you and those that drain you
- Times of the day when you feel more creative or focused

Here we are tracking how different foods, sleep patterns and social interactions affect you. This phase helps you to distinguish between what reflects your true nature and what may be the result of biological imbalance. You may discover, for example, that you feel creative in the evenings but have been forcing yourself to work hard in the mornings because of a rigid work schedule; or that you thrive in deep, meaningful conversations rather than in large social gatherings.

Step 3: Respect your natural rhythms

It is important to understand your biology and to work with it. If you are naturally an introvert, stop forcing yourself to be the life of the party. If you are a night owl, do not make important decisions at 7am. If you have a need for novelty, build variety into your daily routine.

There is a genuinely liberating feeling when this alignment takes place. For example, Gabriel, an investment banker I met years ago, had a genetic disposition towards morning productivity, thrived on routine and craved intellectual challenge, but his work as an investment banker pushed him into late nights, unpredictable schedules and repetitive work. Once he aligned his lifestyle with his biology, transformation became effortless. He eventually launched a successful consultancy firm, crafting a routine that supported his natural strengths and stabilised his energy.

Step 4: Experiment with enhancement

Once you understand your baseline, you can strategically improve your capabilities. Improvement may involve supplements, specific exercise patterns or environmental adjustments that support your natural strengths while factoring in your natural limitations.

Someone with lower baseline dopamine signalling may benefit from strength training, cold exposure or achievement-based goals to increase motivation and drive. Someone with a higher inflammatory baseline may experience a greater shift through an anti-inflammatory diet, stress-management strategies and appropriate supplementation. The key is learning to work with your biology rather than against it.

For the authentic self to emerge, you must recognise that authenticity is not a destination but a way of moving through life. It is the natural expression of your biological design, aligned with your deepest values and dreams. When you live in accordance with your biology, your daily choices begin to match the way evolution shaped your body and mind to function. Transformation then ceases to be a struggle and instead begins to feel like coming home.

Take-home messages

- **You are not broken.** Often, biology is signalling strain rather than a fixed defect. What we often call personality is frequently biology under strain. Research shows that disrupted sleep, rising inflammation, nutrient deficiencies and hormonal shifts can distort mood, clarity and even identity. Support the body, and stability and clarity return. You don't need a new self – you need the conditions that restore access to the self already there.

- **Aligning your biology makes change possible and sustainable.** You cannot willpower your way into a more authentic life if your physiology is pulling in the opposite direction. When the foundations that shape mood, energy, sleep and stress are stabilised, change stops feeling like discipline and starts feeling like alignment – less like hard work and more like returning to your natural state.
- **Mind and body are inseparable.** When both are supported, your true self becomes clear. Modern neuroscience shows thoughts and emotions aren't abstract; they're embodied. When your physiology is steady rather than overwhelmed, your inner world settles too. Authenticity isn't forced – it emerges naturally when mind and body work together.

Once you recognise the forces that have shaped you – your biology, your upbringing, your unconscious patterns – you can begin to sense who you should become rather than reinforcing who you are now or forcing unnatural changes. Identity creates direction, but goals create movement. The next chapter shows you how to anchor that new identity into a path your brain and body can follow.

TWO
Identifying Your Goals

A goal is not just simply something you desire; it is a biological process. When the goal is clear, your brain can mobilise energy towards it more effectively. When the goal is vague, your brain is likely to default to old, familiar behaviours. This is why goal setting is not only a psychological exercise but also a biological one.

David came in to see me. He was an entrepreneur who had built three successful businesses but didn't feel fulfilled. Despite his external signs of success – the fancy house and property portfolio, a comfortable bank balance, and recognition within his professional and social worlds – something was missing. His overriding aspiration? 'I want to be happy.'

When I asked what his goals were, his answer betrayed the issue he was facing:

> 'For the last fifteen years, I have been hunting what success was supposed to look like. I created companies because that is what ambitious entrepreneurs do. I pursued revenue and profit because that is what everyone praised. Now that I have done what I thought I wanted, though, I feel empty. Every morning, I wake up asking myself, *What am I doing?* I had achieved all that I thought I wished to, and yet I am in a place which feels like someone else's life. I no longer even know what I want and why. I have forgotten what really matters to me as I was so trained in what is considered to be important.'

I see this frequently with high achievers who have achieved material success but find themselves without deeper answers regarding purpose and satisfaction. They have become experts at fulfilling external expectations while becoming alienated from their true passions and values. David's situation illustrated a fundamental flaw in how we approach goal setting and achievement. We are so busy climbing the ladder that we fail to check whether it is leaned against the right wall.

We have bought into the concept promoted by the self-help industry that to set a goal we only need to think positively and visualise success. This method was popularised by Hill (1937) in *Think and Grow Rich* almost a century ago and has been repackaged repeatedly as similar methods in several books over the years. While compelling on paper, my work with patients across all walks of life has shown me that effective goal setting requires an understanding of biology and emotions, not just of psychology.

David's desire for happiness reflected a more profound confusion about what he did want out of life. He had worked tirelessly for decades, like so many high achievers, pursuing the goals others told him were most significant, never contemplating if these goals aligned with his own deeper values and biological needs. His success felt hollow because it was not genuinely rooted in his authentic self. He had climbed an entire mountain of achievements only to discover it was not the mountain for him. His desire for happiness was not a true goal but a signal – a sign of mismatch between the life he had built and the one his biology and values were trying to motivate him towards.

To understand why clarity matters so deeply, and why misaligned goals can feel draining, confusing or meaningless, we must turn briefly to the brain's motivation system.

The neuroscience of goal setting

Let's start with dopamine, the key neurotransmitter for goal-driven behaviour in your brain, and one of the primary biological drivers of motivation. As shown in contemporary dopamine research (Lembke 2021), dopamine rises before we reach a goal – during anticipation rather than achievement.

While this pattern mirrors what we see in addiction, where the anticipation of reward often drives behaviour more strongly than the reward itself, ordinary anticipation-driven motivation can be a healthy and adaptive system rather than a pathological one.

Dopamine contributes to this effect, although addiction involves several interacting systems, including opioid-, glutamate- and inhibitory-control circuits. Consider gambling: the possibility of a win triggers a significantly greater dopamine surge than the win itself. Over time, the brain becomes increasingly stimulated by the anticipation rather than the reward. When the reward finally arrives, dopamine drops quickly, making the high fade almost instantly.

This same dynamic applies to our everyday goals, though we rarely recognise it. When we set a goal, whether, for example, losing weight, building a business or mastering piano scales, our brain releases dopamine simply by envisioning success. This initial rush can feel energising and motivating, but if we are not careful, we can become overly attached to the anticipation rather than engaging with the work required to achieve anything meaningful.

The key is learning to derive satisfaction from the work itself – the daily practice, the incremental progress, the skills we develop – rather than fixating on a future moment of arrival and chasing an end point that may never feel as satisfying as the anticipation. Goals that align with our genuine values trigger a natural, sustainable motivation rather than the highs of fantasy. This explains why some goals instantly energise us while others feel like effortful tasks. Think of it like the difference between a stable, satisfying relationship and a volatile one that swings between highs and lows. The former sustains us; the latter leaves us exhausted.

Without genuine interest, motivation relies solely on willpower, a finite resource that inevitably runs out. As Lembke (2021) explains in *Dopamine Nation*, what we truly crave is not the reward itself but the anticipation of it. This ancient survival mechanism once ensured our ancestors continued searching for food, shelter and mates even after temporarily satisfying those needs. Today, however, in a world of constant stimulation and instant gratification, the same system can work against us.

When goals are driven by external pressures – cultural expectations, family or social comparison – dopamine spikes during fantasies of success but quickly collapses once the goal is achieved, leaving satisfaction muted and fleeting. By contrast, when goals are aligned with intrinsic values, motivation becomes steadier, the work itself energising, and the sense of fulfilment deepens. Neurologically, this reflects sustainable engagement: the brain rewards the process, not just the outcome, creating motivation that lasts rather than spikes and fades.

HEAL goals: A sound approach

The business world is in love with SMART goals – ones that are specific, measurable, achievable, relevant and time-bound. While this model provides some order, it often overlooks the biological, psychological and emotional elements of human motivation.

I have worked with many patients and helped them create real and sustainable change, and I now prefer the HEAL framework:

- **H – Health-aligned.** Goals must not be detrimental to your health or that of others. When goals undermine physical wellbeing, they are rarely sustainable.
- **E – Energy-generating.** The pursuit of a goal should energise you rather than deplete you. While ambitious goals might be challenging to achieve, if they reflect your real values, they become invigorating rather than draining.
- **A – Action-inspired.** Goals need to resonate with you and not just be based on expectations from others. External validation might sustain motivation temporarily, but it cannot deliver lasting change.

- **L – Life-integrated.** Goals should integrate naturally into your life rather than requiring you to neglect other priorities. Sustainable goals enhance wellbeing across relationships, health and personal growth rather than forcing you to sacrifice one for another.

HEAL goals support wellbeing during achievement, not only once the goal is completed.

Let me tell you about Mark, a forty-five-year-old workaholic executive, who came to me with full-blown burnout caused by his 'work harder, do more' mentality. His approach to goal setting undermined his health, drained his energy and was motivated by fear rather than authentic desire.

We revised Mark's goals to focus on sustainable performance rather than maximum output. Instead of working longer hours, he committed to maximising his energy through proper sleep, improved nutrition and stress management. Instead of pursuing every opportunity, he became selective, engaging only in projects that genuinely resonated and were aligned with his values and abilities.

The result? His earnings increased and tension decreased. His relationships improved. More importantly, he also regained some work-related enthusiasm that had lured him as a young man into his discipline. His ambitions were finally aligned within the HEAL model. This is how he was able to accomplish more with less effort, and this is what constitutes sustainable success.

The biological reality of motivation

As discussed in Chapter One, biological stability shapes who we can become. Here we turn to how it also shapes what goals we can sustainably pursue.

Traditional goal-setting advice fails because it ignores the fact that your ability to pursue goals is directly related to how you feel physically. My first line of investigations, when patients present struggling with motivation, is to examine key biological factors:

1. Blood sugar levels
2. Hormone homeostasis
3. Sleep
4. Nutrient deficiencies

1. Blood sugar levels

Erratic glucose levels lead to significant energy crashes that make pursuing goals almost impossible. The brain requires 20–25% of the body's glucose (Goyal and Raichle, 2018), and when blood sugar becomes unstable, mental performance and willpower deteriorate quickly. I have seen patients regain their motivation after stabilising their blood glucose through proper nutrition timing.

Take Sarah, a busy working mum who was finding it difficult to keep on top of her healthy eating. Once she simply added protein to every meal, her post-lunch crashes disappeared and she stopped abandoning her plans to go to the gym. A single nutritional adjustment made her goals feel achievable instead of overwhelming.

2. Hormone homeostasis

Hormonal imbalances do not only affect how you feel; they can also directly undermine your capacity to pursue goals.

Hormonal balance is fundamental for sustaining motivation. For example:

- In both men and women, clinically low testosterone can reduce motivation, drive and goal-directed behaviour. Testosterone is just one of many biological factors – alongside neurotransmitters, stress hormones and other endocrine signals – that interact to influence motivation.
- Dysfunction of the thyroid, which regulates your body's metabolic rate, can leave you feeling mentally foggy and physically drained.

- Chronic stress leads to cortisol dysregulation, impairing your ability to make decisions and persist through challenges.

These imbalances can create a destructive cycle – when hormones are dysregulated, your ability to pursue goals is weakened, and the resulting lack of progress and accomplishment increases stress, which in turn further disrupts your hormonal system.

Testosterone has become the flagship of the modern wellness movement, especially among men seeking to reclaim their edge and vitality. In recent years this single hormone has dominated cultural narrative, with podcasts, Instagram accounts and wellness gurus promoting it as the silver bullet to all male malaise. Step into any gym, flick through fitness content online or attend a wellness seminar, and you'll encounter bold claims that boosting testosterone will transform you into an unstoppable force of nature.

The fixation on testosterone, while understandable, represents a dangerous oversimplification of human biology. Although low testosterone can diminish motivation, considering testosterone supplements as a cure-all ignores the complex interaction of hormones, lifestyle factors and physiological elements that truly determine our wellbeing. Men spend thousands of pounds on testosterone replacement therapy, only to remain frustrated when they fail to address their poor sleep, chronic stress, inflammatory diet or the deeper disconnect between their goals and their authentic values. It is like turning up one instrument when the whole orchestra is out of tune.

Real hormonal optimisation may be appropriate for clinically confirmed deficiency, but there is no universal solution. Careful medical supervision and a holistic approach are required to identify underlying causes rather than masking symptoms with supplementation.

Sixty-five-year-old retiree Robert could not understand why, after turning forty, he had become demotivated. Investigations revealed low testosterone and vitamin D levels and also fragmented sleep due to previously unrecognised sleep apnoea. Once these issues were addressed, his motivation returned. He opened a consulting business, trained for marathons and started learning Spanish – things he previously couldn't have imagined.

3. Sleep

Just as sleep shapes identity, the restoration gained through sufficient sleep also determines your capacity for motivation. Without this restoration, even small goals can feel exhausting.

Sleep deprivation undermines cognitive function and emotional regulation, leaving you mentally foggy and emotionally volatile, tricking your mind into thinking everything is tougher. In the case of chronic sleep deprivation, with consistently fewer than six or seven hours per night over weeks or months, the prefrontal cortex – the brain area governing goal seeking and impulse regulation – shows reduced activity and impaired connectivity with emotional centres of the brain (Krause et al, 2017). This impairment manifests as weakened willpower, difficulty maintaining focus on long-term goals, and a tendency towards impulsive decisions that prioritise immediate gratification over sustained effort.

Clinically, people with consistent sleep schedules almost always show stronger goal persistence and less susceptibility to distraction than those living in a chronic sleep deficit.

4. Nutrient deficiencies

The same biochemical gaps that cloud self-understanding also blunt motivation. When the body lacks what it needs, the mind cannot sustain the pursuit of meaningful goals.

Deficiencies in, among others, B vitamins, magnesium, omega-3s and vitamin D impact mood, energy and cognitive function, all of which shape your capacity to pursue goals. These nutrients function as cofactors to produce neurotransmitters and for cellular energy metabolism.

Jennifer, a marketing director, was feeling unmotivated and foggy when she came to me. After conducting thorough testing, we found that despite her seemingly clean diet, Jennifer gained low scores across multiple vitamins and minerals. Once we corrected these deficiencies, with selected supplementation and dietary modifications, she regained clarity and was able to work on goals she had given up on.

Goal hierarchy: Foundations first

Throughout my work with people across vastly different circumstances, I have noticed a consistent pattern. Those who thrive tend to follow an intuitive structure in how they approach goals – a natural order in which the body and mind support ambition. They may not even know it, but their goals align with their basic human needs in a sequential order, as outlined in the table below.

We usually seek to pursue the goals on levels 4 and 5 while neglecting those on levels 1, 2 and 3. This is like attempting to construct an apartment complex on a substandard foundation – it might function in the short term, but it will be fundamentally unstable and eventually collapse.

I worked with Catherine, a non-profit director who thought she was supposed to save the world, and that this would require complete self-sacrifice. She was working a seventy-hour week, eating badly and not exercising, and she had no meaningful relationships

Wellbeing level	*Human needs*
1. Biological foundation	Health and vitality Safety and security Basic needs satisfaction
2. Psychological stability	Emotional regulation Mental clarity Stress management
3. Social connection	Meaningful relationships Community belonging Love and intimacy
4. Personal growth	Skill development Creative expression Self-actualisation
5. Contribution	Service to others Legacy creation Meaning making

outside work. Her desire to change the world was noble, but it was consuming her. She was heading towards burnout, physically exhausted, emotionally isolated and rapidly unable to do the work she cared so deeply about.

We needed to build Catherine's foundation before she could make sustainable impact in her everyday work. This included introducing a consistent sleep pattern, incorporating regular movement in her day, developing skills to regulate her emotions and creating social connections outside work. At first Catherine resisted these suggestions. She felt guilty shifting her focus onto herself when there was so much need in the world. As her health and fitness improved, though, so did her effectiveness. She became more creative, more resilient and more inspirational to her team. The scale of the impact she had within her organisation increased as she adopted a healthier, more sustainable approach to service. By building a strong foundation and then honouring the goal hierarchy, she was able to achieve far more than she had before with significantly less effort and without damaging her health.

The energy equation

All goals come at an energy price, and we all have finite energy. On its surface this is simple, but many people treat energy as infinite and wonder why they are breaking down so often. I remind patients that our energy is like money in a bank account. It is limited, no matter how rich we may be, and the key is to generate wealth as well as to learn how to deploy it effectively.

This is where the flow from Chapter One continues. The same biological limitations that shape identity also shape what you can sustainably chase. Every goal has an energy cost. Motivation without energy is impossible.

When I counsel patients, I try to get them to conceptualise energy as consisting of three types:

1. Physical energy
2. Mental energy
3. Emotional energy

1. Physical energy

This is the easiest to understand, and it boils down to sleep, nutrition, fitness, rest and recovery. It also refers to your general exercise proficiency, which includes your cardiovascular fitness and muscular endurance. Physical energy is relatively reliable – feed your body, sleep well and exercise frequently, and you have a baseline that usually works.

2. Mental energy

This is where things become more complicated. There is only so much mental energy you have, and it gets used every time you make a decision, solve a problem or learn something. It is like the petrol in a car; you might start with a full tank, but every mental task uses fuel. All day your brain makes decisions – which route to take to work, the best way to word that tricky email, whether you should avoid a meeting, what tasks to address first, and so on. That is why a person can be stellar at solving complex problems during prime cognitive time and then, after they have exhausted their mental energy, they become utterly incapable of making even simple decisions.

You need to identify when your own mental energy peaks, ie whether you are a morning person who wakes up feeling quick and sharp or are most productive at night, and then time the hardest parts of your cognitive work accordingly. Your peak performance windows work specifically for you. The decisions that matter should be timed to hit these personal schedule highs, not around when the world thinks you ought to get work done.

3. Emotional energy

This is the most overlooked kind of energy and, in my opinion, the hardest to understand. Although *emotional energy* is not a clinical term, the phenomenon it describes is consistent with the cumulative strain I see repeatedly in clinical practice, when a person chronically suppresses authentic emotional responses. Emotional energy is not just about feeling low or overwhelmed. When your inner values and outer commitments are chronically misaligned, emotional exhaustion accelerates slowly and subtly, and in ways you might not immediately recognise.

Think of the exhaustion that comes with having to silence yourself, forcibly smiling during meetings when your values are being compromised or dismissed, or dealing with relationships that require you to perform in ways that feel unnatural to you. When your inner values and external expectations clash, your emotional energy depletes rapidly.

One patient described this to me as 'drowning in plain sight'. The outside world sees only functionality, while you feel unable to breathe due to a heavy layer of misalignment. You can be physically tired, which rest can cure; or mentally fatigued, which can usually be restored with a healthy meal and a good night's sleep. Emotional depletion runs at a much deeper level, though. It manifests as waking up each day feeling like a stranger to yourself. The insidious nature of emotional drain is that it can leave you exhausted quicker than any physical workout or mental strain ever will, yet it often goes completely unnoticed.

All your sustainable goals should energise you rather than drain you. They should either generate more energy than they consume or fit within your existing energy level, without forcing you to neglect other important areas of your life.

Esther was a working mother who wanted to start a business while also maintaining her corporate job and caring for her family. After getting home from the office and feeding the kids, she spent hours every night collecting data and developing her business plan. She was convinced that if she just worked harder and pushed through the exhaustion, one day her ambitions would come true. She would finally be able to quit her unfulfilling job, her relationship with her husband would become less strained, and the many changes she envisioned would fall into place.

This was a well-intentioned plan on her part, but it completely disregarded her energy balance. Due to the combination of her lack of physical activity, poor nutrition and sleep deprivation, she crashed, creating a significant overall physical energy deficit. While her reduced physical energy might ordinarily have been replenished over the weekend, this rarely happened. She was already experiencing mental strain from the constant decision-making demands at work and had no emotional energy reserves left. She could not even recall the last real moment of intimacy with her husband.

We did not add anything to her already burdened schedule. We first subtracted energy drains and then added new habits to enable the goal of the business she desired. We developed healthier boundaries for Esther at work, better sleep hygiene, and a series of habits to lower the daily cognitive load of decision-making.

Esther's thoughts incrementally became clearer. The final piece of the puzzle was in setting up her business properly, with realistic budgeting and her husband's support, and she achieved freedom and flexibility from unnecessary distractions. The turning point was recognising that energy, not time, was the true bottleneck.

The authenticity filter

When a patient shares a goal with me, one of the most potent questions I ask is whether they would still pursue that goal if no one else would ever know about it, that is, if they were not allowed to tell anybody and received no external recognition or validation.

This is how you can differentiate between real goals and externally influenced goals. True goals energise you because of their congruence with your inner values. They feel powerful and move in a natural flow, where effort no longer feels like work; they become an expression of who you are. For a goal to be truly sustainable, it must activate the brain's reward system in a consistent manner rather than through the intense, short-lived dopamine highs characteristic of compulsive behaviours.

Externally mandated goals drain your energy because you are forcing yourself to go against your natural tendencies and suppress your true self. When you are pursuing goals misaligned with your nature and core values, whether imposed by society or by family, you create tremendous internal conflict. Your logical mind pushes you towards the goal, but deep down you remain acutely aware of the misalignment.

Coping with this internal conflict is exhausting. Your nervous system remains in a state of subtle but persistent anxiety, giving a quiet signal of internal conflict.

I have worked with lawyers who attended law school to please their parents, doctors who studied medicine for social status rather than because of a calling to heal, entrepreneurs who built companies for external validation while despising the work and their role. In every case, achieving these goals left these people feeling hollow. They had succeeded by someone else's standards, not their own.

The authenticity filter also exposes how we are conditioned by culture and family to avoid what should come naturally. Through this exercise Tom, a successful lawyer, discovered that he had never wanted a career in law. His father was a lawyer, so Tom had followed the same script. He was a natural teacher and felt drawn to working with young people. His high-achieving family had always dismissed teaching as impractical, but Tom was quickly filled with energy when he began to follow his true calling. Even though he was making less money, he felt richer because his work aligned with his values. His relationships improved as he was no longer harbouring the bitterness of disappointed dreams. Perhaps most surprisingly, as the chronic stress of feeling a fraud lifted, his body healed.

Practical goal design

Whether patients consult me with clear goals or come needing to identify them, I guide them through a process that addresses their biological makeup alongside critical psychological and emotional insights:

- **Biology assessment.** Before any goal can be pursued, you need a strong physical foundation from which to launch meaningful goals. When you are constantly exhausted, your hormones are dysregulated or you have nutrient deficiencies, there is little chance of making meaningful progress. This step includes assessment of sleep quality, energy patterns, stress responses and basic health markers.

- **Energy audit.** Here we examine to what you currently dedicate your physical, mental and emotional energy. The reality for many of us is that we spend a considerable amount of time on activities that don't align with our values or beliefs. This audit identifies opportunities for redirection rather than addition.
- **Values clarification.** This is crucial though challenging work. Through a series of exercises, you gain clarity on what truly matters to you (versus what you are 'supposed' to care about). It means confronting family expectations and cultural pressures, and not comparing yourself to others. Values clarification is not an intellectual exercise; it is an embodied process. You discover which goals energise you and which deplete you by tuning into your body's responses, not through logical analysis alone.
- **Goal hierarchy.** Next we map goals against the hierarchy described earlier, meaning you must address foundation-related goals before moving on to higher aspirations. This approach avoids the

common error of building ambitious objectives on unstable foundations, which often leads to failure.

- **Integration planning.** In this final stage we create a sustainable plan for achieving your goals without compromising your health, relationships or overall wellbeing. This includes energy management strategies, appropriate support systems, and built-in flexibility to maintain balance as circumstances change.

The compound effect of aligned goals

Magic happens when your goals are naturally aligned with your:

- Biology
- Psychology
- Emotions
- Authentic values

The pursuit of aligned goals becomes energising rather than requiring constant willpower and motivation, and the goals improve other areas of your life instead of competing with them. I call this alignment *sustainable passion* – the profound fulfilment that arises when living from your true nature and serving noble aims. This is not always easy to achieve.

One of my patients was Neville, a forty-something Lebanese man with many physical complaints, who brooded on deep inner turmoil. Over the course of a few sessions, he took a deep breath and verbalised his struggle with his sexual identity. He admitted that he felt like a square peg in a round hole, the latter representing his deeply traditional family and community, where revealing his sexuality could result in alienation. Instead of me telling him to abandon his cultural roots or confront them, we developed a process that I refer to as *authentic navigation* – a way for him to honour himself and also his culture.

The many words of wisdom Neville had heard over the years melted into a single goal of learning to trust himself and loving himself more, while building a space safe enough for him to take off his mask. This meant building supportive connections, contributing to causes he cared about and choosing who he could safely confide in.

The goals ticked every facet of the HEAL framework:

- **Health-aligned** – supporting his mental health by eliminating a painful burden
- **Energy-generating** – creating energy through meaningful connection and service, aligned with his sense of purpose
- **Action-inspired** – pursuing what genuinely mattered to him, not what others expected

- **Life-integrated** – honouring his deeper values of compassion and family loyalty

Three years later Neville realised that he had become immensely resilient and found ways to be himself within his constraints. By learning to honour his heritage while remaining genuine, he quietly became an advocate for others in similar positions. He did this in such a way that his cultural history and his true self could all exist safely in the same place.

His experience showed me that pursuing your best-aligned goals does not have to involve burning bridges or hurting others. Sometimes the greatest change comes from the gradual unfolding of intentional honesty. When a goal is authentic and aligned with the way biology works (rather than with family or social pressures), it moves rapidly from being exhausting to feeling sustainable. Moreover, the achievement of such goals is rewarding in the long run, as it leads to fulfilment rather than empty accomplishment. Progress becomes self-sustaining rather than draining.

Emotional harmony – the musical analogy

I often tell patients that, just as there are seven natural musical notes that can be combined in many ways, we each have a repertoire of emotional responses that can be harmoniously arranged or randomly scattered. Link emotions together in a logical response to appropriate situations, and you create a melody – life as an ensemble.

We can all be trained to identify our emotions and connect them in a balanced manner with specific situations. As we respond to the experiences of life with the appropriate emotion – curiosity over anger when trying something new, gratitude over expectation when help is offered, compassion over judgement when faced with another's suffering – we make a symphony in our soul which makes pursuing our goals feel far less arduous and more enduring.

Just remember that your goals are not only destinations but also the blueprints of your daily life. Choose goals that align with your authentic nature rather than ones that force you to struggle against who you truly are, and the process of achieving them will be as enriching as the accomplishment.

Never forget, it is not your mission to be somebody else. It is about becoming who you are, informed by goals that respect both your biology and your most fervent hopes. Once all is aligned, transformation no longer feels like becoming anything other than your essence, supporting what deeply matters to you.

Take-home messages

- **Motivation isn't the issue – biological fit is.** Dopamine drives the high of anticipation rather than of achievement. That's why some goals feel exhilarating at first but quickly fade. When a goal reflects cultural pressure or imported expectations, your biology won't invest in it. What looks like a motivation problem is really a mismatch – your biology simply cannot sustain a goal that isn't truly your own.

- **Energy determines what you can sustain, so we need to budget it wisely.** Physical, mental and emotional energy are limited resources. Goals that continually drain you tend to collapse, and even when achieved, they can leave you feeling hollow. Sustainable goals fit your real capacity and replenish your reserves over time. Learning to budget your energy is far more important than managing your time.
- **The HEAL framework supports progress that lasts.** Goal setting using the HEAL framework supports wellbeing throughout the journey, not only at the finish line. When goals are designed to work with your biology rather than against it, progress feels steadier, more meaningful and sustainable, and never forced.

You can set extraordinary goals, but if your physiology is depleted, dysregulated or overwhelmed, your best intentions collapse under the weight of biology. To pursue a life that inspires you and resonates with you, your body must have the energy, resilience and internal chemistry to sustain that pursuit. That is why the next chapter turns to physical health – the engine of every transformation.

THREE

Identifying Your Health: The Physical, Foundation-Creating Health

A confession to you first: my medical training was based largely on how to treat symptoms, with little regard for prevention or for enhancing health. I always sensed prevention should be medicine's focus, yet throughout my training, the priority was on treating illness rather than on promoting health.

When she first came to my office, sixty-seven-year-old Mrs Patterson walked in with a plastic bag filled with seventeen medications, for hypertension, diabetes, arthritis, depression, insomnia and more. Specialists had prescribed a pill for each condition. She opened her worn eyes and told me, 'Doctor, I just feel like I am dying slowly, and all these medicines are supposed to make me better.'

That moment altered how I wanted to practise medicine and revealed just how much our health system prioritises disease management, while gradually overlooking the creation and protection of health itself. It also became clear to me that the life-changing transformations celebrated in countless self-help books are impossible without first establishing physical health.

Let me be clear: I am not dismissing modern medicine and joining ranks with those who claim positive thinking alone can replace medical care, and I am not siding with those that demonise all pharmaceutical treatments. My clinical experience has shown me too often how dangerous such oversimplification can be.

Walk the paediatric wards of any hospital and you will meet children who radiate more vitality and hope than many healthy adults. Kids who dream big, laugh with abandon and remain genuinely hopeful, even while battling serious conditions like leukaemia, cystic fibrosis or heart defects. These extraordinary young people remind us that a positive mindset alone cannot overcome serious illness. Hope and resilience matter immensely for quality of life and treatment adherence, but without medical intervention, even the most positive outlook has its limits. We need both: the power of a positive mind, combined with medical intervention.

It is extraordinary how far modern medicine has come. Antenatal care reduces maternal deaths, insulin keeps diabetics alive, surgical techniques manage to spare hearts that would otherwise deteriorate, and antibiotics are sometimes the difference between life and death. My own grandfather died, long before I was born, of septicaemia from a tiny blister caused by new shoes. If he had had access to the antibiotics we have now, this trivial injury would not have taken his life, and I might have known him.

This chapter is not an argument against medicine but a call to rebalance it, to place health creation alongside disease treatment.

I am not calling for an earthy nirvana of meditation and wheatgrass smoothies. What I am suggesting is infinitely vast. It's about deep appreciation for what medical interventions can offer but with the realisation that our current system is too orientated towards disease management, with insufficient focus on the early prevention of disease.

The prevention revolution

Positive thinking and willpower alone cannot compensate for poor physical health. Your body is not merely a vessel for your mind; it's the foundation of all change.

In my practice I have seen prisoners who changed their lives more dramatically than billionaires with all the wealth in the world. The difference was not motivation or privilege; it was that prisoners understood the need to address their physical foundation first.

Think about research from the blue zones, those extraordinary communities where people habitually reach the age of 100. The work of Buettner (2008) and his discoveries in these communities have shown us something major: none of these places focus on treating disease. Their lifestyle patterns are associated with a delay onset and, in some cases, prevention of many age-related diseases.

Let me share what inspired me most when I discovered these communities. I expected the secret to lie in sophisticated medical interventions, hidden supplements and cutting-edge treatments. What I found, however, was so beautifully simple that it challenged everything I'd previously understood about health and longevity.

I have been told about ninety-year-old fishermen on the island of Ikaria in Greece who, strong in body and mind, still dive for sponges. There is no pharmaceutical secret. They walk uphill to their gardens, take siestas aligned to their circadian rhythms and enjoy evening gatherings that unite three generations for meals and storytelling. These are not health interventions; they are simply how life is lived.

In the high mountain villages in Sardinia, I witnessed something else that challenged my assumptions about ageing. Farmers in their eighties and nineties still tended sheep on steep terrain, naturally preserving muscle mass and bone density through functional movement. No gym membership, no structured programmes – just lives that required movement.

For me the most impressive discovery was the relationship these communities enjoy with food. In Loma Linda in California, land of the Seventh-day Adventists, families gather for plant-rich meals and stop eating at around 80% fullness, not as a dietary technique but as cultural wisdom. Food represents connection, tradition and joy.

We don't need to try to imitate any specific community. The deeper lesson is that prevention is not mystical or complicated – it is the accumulation of simple, repeatable daily behaviours that protect health long before disease arrives. In clinical practice I see that prevention looks less like strict programmes and far more like ordinary choices: walking as part of daily life, eating food that resembles its natural form, nurturing relationships, sleeping with some regularity and managing stress before it turns into chronic inflammation. These habits, practised consistently, create the biological environment in which disease struggles to take hold.

The centenarians in Okinawa, Japan, showed me how *ikigai,* one's sense of purpose, supports longevity. Elderly women tend their gardens not because a doctor has prescribed activity but because their families and communities need vegetables. They do not pursue longevity; they live in ways that make longevity a consequence.

Okinawans also practise *hara hachi bu* – a habit that likely contributes to metabolic health and improved insulin sensitivity and may support cellular 'cleanup' processes such as autophagy under caloric restriction conditions, although this has not been directly confirmed in humans. Eating slowly and paying attention to hunger cues are things we can all learn.

What fundamentally separated my doctor self from my human self was realising that these people are not trying to live to 100. This recognition forced me to confront an uncomfortable truth about modern medicine: we excel at treating disease, yet we are far less skilled at creating health. Much of what we do medically could be prevented if we embraced basic principles of human living.

The blue zones taught me that longevity does not come from prescriptions or strict protocols. It emerges from daily choices, aligned with human biology, as we navigate life's challenges. These communities have not discovered some secret fountain of youth; they have maintained lifestyle patterns consistent with the fundamentals of wellbeing.

Reflecting on my patients, I realised that those who improved most didn't always have the best healthcare. They were the ones whose daily lives naturally included movement, purpose, community contact, simple food and stress regulation. This is why I am obsessed with prevention over intervention. It is why I believe your everyday choices can influence your genetics far more than people imagine. It is also where my faith lies – not in a silver bullet of advanced science but in meeting the basic human needs that transcend time and culture.

The blue zones suggest that health often emerges from living in ways aligned with basic human needs rather than through strain or hypervigilance. It arises when we stop fighting our biology and start living in alignment with it. This is *the* foundation on which lasting personal change must stand – not in the grand pursuit of becoming better but in adopting small and repeated actions that create an environment where the highest self can emerge naturally, just as it has done for generations in the blue zones' remarkable, long-living communities.

The inflammation epidemic

Allow me to introduce you to a silent epidemic that is affecting millions. It is thought to be widespread in industrialised societies, although exact prevalence varies depending on how inflammation is defined. Still, very few people even realise it's there.

You do not feel inflammation, but you feel its consequences, which can make personal growth essentially impossible in five main areas:

1. Arteries
2. Cognitive decline
3. Depressive and anxiety symptoms
4. Energy
5. Willpower

1. Arteries

A large body of scientific research shows that, over time, chronic inflammation promotes plaque formation and calcification within the arteries contributing to cardiovascular events such as heart attack and stroke. Inflammatory processes damage the endothelial lining of blood vessels, making them less elastic and less efficient at regulating blood flow. This impairs the delivery of oxygen and nutrients to tissues throughout the body, including the brain.

As arterial health declines, so does overall physiological resilience. Reduced vascular efficiency places greater strain on the heart, limits physical stamina and subtly undermines cognitive performance by restricting cerebral blood flow. Even before overt cardiovascular disease develops, low-grade inflammation can diminish exercise tolerance, slow recovery and increase fatigue, eroding the physical capacity required to sustain effort over time. In this way, vascular inflammation does not only threaten long-term health; it directly constrains day-to-day energy, focus and the ability to pursue goals consistently.

2. Cognitive decline

Inflammatory cytokines cross over from the blood into the brain, causing you to feel foggy or to lose focus on what you are doing.

Research led by Miller (2009) at Emory University has found that inflammatory cytokines, especially interleukin-1β (IL-1β), tumour necrosis factor-α (TNF-α) and interleukin-6 (IL-6), can infiltrate the blood–brain barrier and also interfere with neurotransmitter function.

In a study by Cohen et al (2003) in the *Journal of Molecular Neuroscience,* healthy volunteers received low-dose endotoxin (0.8 ng/kg of Salmonella endotoxin) for mild inflammation. There were significant effects on declarative memory, lasting at least nine hours after administration, yet the study showed no association with the inflammatory markers level or serum cortisol. Similar studies with other endotoxins have shown that even minor inflammatory changes such as those following vaccination can prompt cognitive deficits, with participants experiencing memory impairments, mood alterations and anxiety. These findings show that systemic inflammation can rapidly induce cognitive deterioration, with effects observable in as little as a few hours after endotoxin administration. Chronic inflammation has been linked to accelerated cognitive decline in several studies (Marsland et al, 2015), highlighting the role of immune signalling in brain ageing.

Research from the Framingham Heart Study by Jefferson et al (2007) found that people with higher levels of inflammation had smaller total brain volumes and performed worse on tests of executive function, ie of cognitive skills needed to set goals, plan and monitor behaviour.

3. Depressive and anxiety symptoms

Inflammation can increase depressive and anxiety symptoms through established biochemical pathways, with mood continuing to deteriorate even after inflammation peaks. This isn't just you psyching yourself out; it's in your blood.

Research conducted by Pariante (2017) at King's College London has identified specific mechanisms through which inflammatory cytokines produce depressive symptoms that overlap with those seen in major depressive disorder.

Inflammatory cytokines activate an enzyme called indoleamine 2,3-dioxygenase (IDO), which breaks down tryptophan, the precursor to serotonin. This reduces your body's ability to produce adequate serotonin, impairing mood regulation. At the same time, this process increases the production of quinolinic acid – a neurotoxin that damages brain cells and generates anxiety symptoms, creating a vicious cycle where inflammation perpetuates itself and impairs mental health.

In practical terms, this means that many people who supposedly feel depressed for no reason might be experiencing a biological state rather than a purely psychological one.

4. Energy

Your body diverts energy to fight inflammation rather than providing fuel for performance and growth. In a state of inflammation your body can effectively enter a wartime economy, repurposing energy and resources from growth, repair and optimal performance to inflammatory processes.

A study by Dantzer (2009) at MD Anderson Cancer Center noted that inflammatory cytokines directly impair mitochondrial function, which produces energy inside your cells. TNF-α and IL-1β can impair mitochondrial efficiency in certain contexts, reducing adenosine triphosphate (ATP) production in ways that contribute to fatigue.

Higher inflammatory markers have been associated with lower motivation to engage in difficult tasks. A study published in the journal *Brain, Behaviour, and Immunity* (Raison and Miller, 2013), found that individuals with elevated inflammation showed reduced motivation when offered monetary rewards for completing challenging tasks. This reduction in motivation is mediated by brain regions like the ventral striatum and ventromedial prefrontal cortex, which are critical for motivation and reward processing. Brain imaging showed decreased activity in these regions when inflammatory markers were elevated.

This is why many people who feel unmotivated may actually be experiencing a biological energy deficit, not a character flaw.

5. Willpower

Willpower is reduced by inflammation that attacks the prefrontal cortex, the home of self-regulation. Research conducted by Eisenberger (2012) at the University of California demonstrated that inflammatory cytokines seek out the prefrontal cortex area, suppressing its function and making it much harder for individuals to self-regulate their actions.

Research by Joyce, et al (2025) demonstrates that inflammatory cytokines directly target the dorsolateral prefrontal cortex, impairing working memory, abstraction and the thoughtful regulation of attention, action and emotion. This research shows how stress and inflammation weaken cognitive control by affecting prefrontal networks that are essential for self-regulation.

I recall working with a forty-two-year-old executive, Arthur, who was reading every productivity book available but could not stick with any of the habits he attempted to develop. His labs confirmed significant signs of inflammation. It was only after working on his sleep, cutting out all processed foods and adding in a few key anti-inflammatory nutrients that he regained mental clarity. Those productivity strategies suddenly worked seamlessly. Rather than a lack of willpower, Arthur's issues had been due to a biological misalignment.

Foundation health markers

You cannot optimise what you do not measure, and without objective data you cannot know if you are improving. Before pursuing any transformation goals, I therefore encourage my patients to establish baseline measurements in these key areas:

- **Metabolic health.** This is your body's ability to efficiently process energy. Poor metabolic health creates energy swings that make consistent behaviour nearly impossible. Ideal rates are:
  - Fasting glucose: 70–85 mg/dL (not the 'normal' range of up to 100)

  - Fasting insulin: Under 5 mIU/L
  - HbA1c: Under 5.5%
  - Triglyceride to high-density lipoprotein ('good' cholesterol) ratio: Under 2.0

  Simply by stabilising their blood sugar, I have witnessed patients become remotivated and regain mental clarity. By exploring her chronobiology and making meaningful modifications in meal timing and composition, Maria, a tired schoolteacher with late-night munchies, finally began to feel some spark for a new burst of life.

- **Inflammatory status.** Chronic inflammation is like having a small fire constantly burning in your body. It is exhausting and makes everything harder. Ideal levels are:
  - C-reactive protein (CRP): Under 1.0 mg/L
  - Erythrocyte sedimentation rate (ESR): Age-appropriate ranges
  - Homocysteine: 6–10 µmol/L
- **Hormonal balance.** Your hormones influence processes related to motivation, mood and physical recovery. Key markers include:
  - Thyroid function: Thyroid-stimulating hormone (TSH), free T3, free T4, reverse T3
  - Sex hormones: Testosterone, oestrogen, progesterone

  - Stress hormones: Cortisol pattern throughout the day
  - Sleep hormones: Melatonin production

- **Cardiovascular fitness.** This is not about looking good; it refers to your body's ability to deliver oxygen and nutrients to your brain and organs.
  - Resting heart rate: Lower is generally better
  - Blood pressure: Optimal is 110/70–120/80
  - VO_2 max (the maximum volume of oxygen your body can consume during intense exercise): Strongly associated with longevity and with better cognitive ageing

- **Body composition.** This goes far beyond weight or the simplistic BMI, which are both crude and often misleading measures.
  - Muscle mass: Essential for metabolic health and ageing
  - Visceral fat: The dangerous fat around organs
  - Bone density: Particularly important as we age

The movement medicine

Let me be blunt: if you are going to transform your life, you have to exercise. Evidence clearly shows exercise is the best intervention for physical and mental health. However, this is where people often go wrong, believing that exercise must be difficult, requires huge amounts of time or involves suffering. Having treated a whole range of patients for all types of health issues, I can assure you that the effective exercise dose for health is surprisingly low.

Movement is the non-negotiable foundation. We are meant to move our bodies. Our ancestors kept active in hunting, gathering, building and farming. The reality of modern sedentary living is a relatively new experiment, the consequences of which are dire for physical, mental and emotional health.

To transform our health through movement, we do not need a gym membership or expensive equipment. Some of the most potent movement interventions are free and available to be done anywhere. Consistency is key, together with an appreciation for how movement literally changes your brain and body.

Consider Maria, a fifty-eight-year-old accountant who struggled with back pain for years and complained of low energy and what she called brain fog. She believed that she needed surgery for her back and medication to combat the fatigue. I told her to start walking for ten minutes after every meal, completing three small walks a day. Within two weeks her mental clarity improved, and she had much less back pain. After one month her energy was up, and she was sleeping much better than she had for years. Her brain fog had also cleared, leading to her being productive at work.

A large study published in the journal *Circulation* (Lee et al, 2022) discovered something that should revolutionise how we think about exercise and health: just 150 minutes of moderate activity per week, about twenty minutes a day – less time than most spend scrolling through social media – is enough to reduce your risk of premature death by 20–30%. If you could take a pill and get these results, pharmaceutical companies would make billions of pounds and this drug would be in the water supply. This 'cure' is available to us all, though – it's as simple as a stroll or an easy bike ride.

There is something even more extraordinary. The difference between being sedentary and walking twenty minutes a day has a bigger impact than the difference between moderate exercise and Olympian training. That means that even if you are deeply sedentary, you can experience the most drastic health upgrade simply by weaving some slow and steady movement into your day. Like compound interest, the earlier in life you start and the more regularly you do this, the greater your net gain will be over time. Even small, consistent efforts accumulate benefits.

The science of how movement heals seems almost magical, yet it is happening in your body right now. As you move, your muscles release myokines, signalling molecules, or 'muscle messages', that travel through your bloodstream acting like an internal pharmacy and supporting your body's functions. These molecules are active chemical messengers that promote healing and regeneration through your entire body.

They increase your insulin sensitivity, which is good for the management of blood sugar and can help you avoid diabetes. They boost immune function, thereby updating the body's natural defence systems. They also stimulate the birth of new brain cells; yes, movement is strongly associated with greater brain resilience and cognitive capacity. At the cellular level, certain myokines have powerful anti-inflammatory effects, without the side effects of medications.

One of the most exciting discoveries in modern neuroscience is that exercise is like Miracle-Gro® for your brain. Each workout rewires, regenerates and changes the structure of your most important organ, as highlighted by Harvard Medical School psychiatrist Ratey (2008). His research highlights how physical activity supercharges the production of a protein, brain-derived neurotrophic factor (BDNF), which acts like brain fertiliser. BDNF is a master gardener for your brain, helping existing neurons survive and thrive in today's toxic environment and causing the growth of new neurons and synapses – a process known as *synaptic plasticity*. This means you can regenerate brain tissue well into old age.

More recent research by Ruiz-González et al (2021), building on Ratey's earlier foundational work, demonstrates that physical exercise interventions can enhance plasma BDNF levels in individuals with neurodegenerative disorders, indicating potential therapeutic benefits for these conditions.

We can produce new brain cells throughout life, primarily in specific brain regions such as the hippocampus, although the rate naturally changes with age and can be enhanced by movement. Every time you move your body, you are quite literally growing new brain cells and building new connections between those neurons. This has a massive implication – that early-morning run doesn't only help make your heart stronger; it also enhances brain development. An afternoon walk does more than burning calories; it also forges new neural pathways that will improve memory, lead to better mood and increase cognitive function.

In short, exercise is the closest thing we have to a miracle drug. It shows the unique promise of counteracting some of the effects of ageing on the brain.

The non-negotiables of exercise

- 150 minutes of moderate cardiovascular activity per week (twenty minutes per day)
- Strength training two or three times per week

- Movement breaks throughout the day if you sit a lot at work

The key is finding movement you enjoy and can maintain, which could be as simple as dancing, gardening or playing with grandkids. The greatest exercise is the one you will do frequently.

Sleep: The ultimate performance enhancer

If there was a single intervention I could give you to improve your health and expedite your transformation, it would be sleep optimisation. Sadly, we treat sleep as a luxury in our productivity-obsessed culture.

What happens when you do not get enough sleep:

- Your self-regulation capacity drops markedly.
- Your memory is impaired.
- Your immune system weakens.
- Your hormones become dysregulated.
- Your metabolism slows down.

I have witnessed individuals' lives fall into place simply by them prioritising sleep. For example, Michael was a startup originator working sixteen-hour days and getting by on four to five hours of sleep each night. He took pride in the 'grind', but his sales were low because he was making poor decisions. Once he committed to getting seven to eight hours of sleep per night, his productivity soared, his mood was better, and he worked more efficiently.

I often explain the importance of sleep to patients by comparing it to how we all religiously charge the batteries of our mobile phones for optimal performance. Why not fully charge your own batteries with the same consistency?

The way to achieve good-quality sleep is to develop a sleep routine that signals to your body and mind that it is time to rest. I like to have my patients think of this as the famous conditioning experiment on dogs carried out by Ivan Pavlov (1927). He found that ringing a bell shortly before feeding his dogs eventually made them salivate when they heard the bell, without them seeing the food. Their minds had been trained to link the bell with being fed. Similarly, we can train our brains to relate sleep with certain activities and environments. After some time, persisting with the same pre-sleep activities every night – for example, taking a warm bath, reducing lighting, reading – your brain associates these actions with rest and begins discharging melatonin, lowering your core temperature and inducing sleep.

Of course, I realise all of us have various real-world issues to contend with and that maintaining perfect sleep hygiene can be challenging. A large part of my career has required me to travel overseas, continuously fighting jet lag and attempting to nap in hotels with dubious blackout curtains and inscrutable temperature settings. I also understand shift work, newborns breaking up sleep, upwardly mobile careers and general chaos sabotaging our health. What I have discovered, though, both as a doctor and from my own personal experience, is that there are realistic, achievable strategies that can help many people dramatically increase their chances of falling and staying asleep at night, no matter how long their workday is or how full of responsibility life has become.

Sleep optimisation protocol

- Consistent sleep and wake times (even on weekends)
- A cool, dark, quiet bedroom environment
- No screens for one to two hours before bed
- Morning light exposure to regulate circadian rhythms
- Limited stimulants, including caffeine and certain medications, after 2pm
- A consistent pre-sleep routine to condition your brain for rest

The nutrition foundation

I will explore nutrition in more depth in Chapter Six, but I need to establish the baseline here, because without adequate fuelling, your brain and body cannot sustain transformation. Poor nutrition creates unpredictable energy fluctuations that make consistent behaviour almost impossible. Stability in blood sugar and micronutrient status is not optional; it is the platform on which motivation, clarity and emotional balance rest.

The basics

- Consume real, whole foods as much as possible.
- Include a source of protein with every meal to stabilise energy and support recovery.
- Stay adequately hydrated throughout the day.
- Time your meals to avoid blood sugar swings, which destabilise mood and focus.
- If testing identifies deficiencies, consider targeted nutrient support rather than generic supplementation.

Nutrition is not about rigid rules or restriction; it is about creating a consistent biological baseline so your body can power the behaviour, decision-making and resilience required for your goals.

Recovery: The missing piece

Many understand that stress drives adaptation and growth. What our achievement-obsessed culture fails to appreciate is that recovery is where the real growth occurs. Without it, stress does not make you stronger; it breaks you down.

During any period of effort – such as lifting weights, learning a new skill or pursuing a challenging project – you are creating micro-damage in your muscles, brain and nervous system. The transformation happens afterwards, during recovery, when your body repairs muscle fibres, consolidates memories, strengthens neural pathways and recalibrates your stress systems.

The difficult part is not the stress itself. It's allowing enough recovery for adaptation to take place. Without recovery, the same stress that normally helps to create progress instead generates fatigue, irritability, impaired cognition and eventual burnout.

To optimise recovery I recommend:

- **Prioritising sleep.** This is when your body repairs tissue, consolidates learning and clears metabolic waste from your brain.
- **Scheduling rest.** It is important to avoid intense exercise every day. It is better to schedule regular breaks, taking at least one or two full rest days per

week and alternating between high-intensity and lower-intensity work.

- **Practising stress-reduction techniques.** These include meditation, slow and deep breathing, and exposure to nature.
- **Eating adequately, including enough protein.** Recovery requires physical building blocks, not just rest.
- **Listening to your body.** Persistent fatigue, irritability, poor sleep or declined performance signal the need for more recovery, not more effort.

Recovery is not indulgence; it is a biological requirement. Without it, you cannot access the benefits of your hard work or sustain your goals.

The physical integration blueprint

Mrs Patterson, who I mentioned at the start of this chapter, provides an ideal case history of what integration looks like. Rather than dealing with her seventeen conditions individually, we worked on addressing the roots of her health issues. We improved her nutrition, kept her moving regularly, helped her get better sleep and encouraged more social behaviour with community involvement. Within six months she was able to stop fourteen of her seventeen medications. Her energy levels increased, and she became more energised, taking on a role in a local literacy programme that she had always desired but had felt too fatigued and defeated to pursue.

This is what I need you to understand: with a solid baseline of physical vitality, almost everything improves – your thinking, creativity, emotional wellbeing and resilience. You gain the energy to go after your goals, the mental clarity to make good decisions and the emotional fortitude to cope with unplanned events.

Do not be fooled into believing you can simply think your way into transformation while ignoring what your body requires. You must begin by making changes in your physical body first; only then will creative possibilities that previously felt out of reach start to feel natural or even joyful.

Your body is *not* your enemy; it is your greatest ally in transformation. If treated with the respect and care it deserves, it will carry you to your highest aspirations. Addressing your physical health is the foundation of any transformation. If you don't have a body that can keep up with you on this journey, you will get stuck. When your biology is aligned, everything else becomes more possible, more sustainable and far less draining.

Take-home messages

- **Inflammation is invisible, but it can prevent transformation.** Low-grade inflammation is common in industrialised societies and quietly disrupts countless psychological, emotional and physical processes. Addressing it through sleep, movement, nutrition and stress reduction is often the first true turning point in restoring wellbeing, long before willpower or mindset can help. In the presence of persistent inflammation, transformation becomes almost impossible.
- **Movement is medicine – just twenty minutes a day can change everything.** As little as twenty minutes of daily movement – less time than most people spend on social media – confers dramatic health benefits. It enhances energy, stabilises mood, supports cognition and initiates biological repair in ways far more potent than most people realise. Consistency matters far more than intensity, and movement alone begins mending the biology every other change relies on.
- **Physical health is your starting point, not an afterthought.** You cannot think, plan or will yourself into change if your body cannot keep up. When sleep, movement, nutrition and recovery are in place, your biology stops resisting you and starts supporting you. With a strong physical base, clarity improves, motivation returns, and the psychological and emotional work of

transformation becomes not only possible but far more natural and joyful.

Strong physical foundations create capacity, but capacity alone doesn't silence anxiety, dissolve old wounds or resolve emotional patterns that hold you back. The body can be thriving while the mind remains exhausted, or vice versa. To truly achieve transformation, physical vitality must be paired with emotional clarity and mental steadiness. Let's see how.

FOUR
Identifying Your Stress: Mental And Emotional Wellness

Every time Frank sobbed in my office is forever etched in my mind. This was a man who had set up a multimillion-pound business, led high-power boardroom meetings and seemingly knew how to handle life. Here he sat, broken and in tears, crying, 'Doctor, I am drowning, and I cannot figure out why.'

In all the ways Frank knew how, and in line with the how-to traditional measures of success, he had done everything 'right'. He regularly worked out, ate perfectly, had flawless blood work and was taking all the right supplements. However, he was plagued by something we seldom talk about: a widespread pattern of mental and emotional dysfunction that is undermining transformation even in those who appear most disciplined.

The system that connects body, mind and emotion

All too often we've treated mental health as the stepchild of illness, as if it were only distantly related to physical health, with the brain somehow disconnected from the body. This is a blind spot in both the medical and personal development worlds – one that continues to hold millions back from experiencing lasting transformation.

When you talk about getting butterflies in your stomach before you deliver a presentation, it's not just a turn of phrase. It's a pretty accurate description of the literal connection between your mind and your gut, known as the digestive system's *second brain.* When you become red-faced with embarrassment, your emotions are causing a physical change in your cardiovascular system. A headache triggered by chronic worry means your mind is having a measurable, physical effect on blood vessels and muscle tension.

Take Erika, a high-powered lawyer who sought my help for supposedly idiopathic chronic fatigue. Several specialists had detected nothing wrong in her blood work, heart or lungs, yet she was struggling to make it through a workday without feeling exhausted. Diagnoses considered by the doctors she had seen included fibromyalgia or chronic fatigue syndrome.

After some time working together, we uncovered three years of pent-up anger following the death of her father. Erika was dealing with this while internally concealing her grief and rage, out of public view. As we started unravelling these emotions through talk therapy and body work, she felt a sudden shift in her energy. The physical and emotional issues weren't distinct from each other; instead, they were different expressions of an integrated system. Containing or suppressing the emotions had been an enormous effort, which had left her body weary.

This raises important questions about the mind–body link. Is our mental state really related to whether our body is functioning properly? How does the immune system shape the brain and mental experience across our lifespan? Might chronic psychological stress influence biological processes and modulate nervous, immune and endocrine functions and gut microbiota?

Research by Bower and Kuhlman (2023) shows that emotional stress triggers biological changes throughout the body, confirming the deep connection between mental and physical health. Building on this, research by Bernad et al (2024) suggests that chronic stress and suppressed emotions can alter gene regulation at multiple levels, including epigenetic mechanisms – chemical modifications that change how genes behave without altering the DNA sequence itself. Their research highlights several key stress-responsive genes involved in emotional regulation, stress resilience and neural plasticity. In plain terms, prolonged emotional strain can change the way your cells operate, influencing mood and affecting immunity and long-term health at a molecular level.

Go back to Pert's (1997) landmark study on neuropeptides we discussed earlier, and you realise why mental health and emotional health are joined at the hip with physical health. Her research showed that emotions are not just abstract concepts in the mind; they are embodied chemical events that spread across your physiology. This means that chronic stress, trauma or negative emotional states not only affect your mood; they also change the biochemistry of every organ system in your body.

Imagine what happens in the case of chronic anxiety or depression. Pert's research shows that the neuropeptides associated with those emotional states can influence immune activity in ways that can promote inflammation and impair healing when stress becomes chronic. By contrast, when you engage in loving relationships, satisfying work or fulfilling activities that evoke positive emotions, you generate physiological changes, including shifts in hormones and immune signalling. This reinforces our understanding of mental and emotional health, shifting them from luxury items to essential building blocks of physical health. The way you feel emotionally isn't just spilling over into the way you think; it's directly affecting how biochemically healthy or unhealthy you are.

Mental and emotional health are deeply important. With growing scientific backing, addressing emotional health is not just a matter of positive thinking or affirmations. It is the act of genuinely considering your feelings as one of the most important indicators of overall vitality and health. What I have observed repeatedly, regardless of whether patients have access to the best psychologists money can buy, is that psychological work alone often cannot fully counteract the biological effects of chronic stress unless the underlying physiology is also addressed.

Princess Nevine had been in therapy for years, working with top psychiatrists and psychologists all over the world. She knew her patterns, was enlightened about the workings of her family system and could talk with psychological sophistication about how anxious she always felt. She was nevertheless plagued by panic attacks and insomnia, and she felt nothing except numbness that medication did not fix. On the surface, as the prototype of the 'modern-day princess', she seemed to have it all, but decades in the fishbowl and feeling caged had begun wreaking havoc on her body. She had high cortisol levels, a severely disrupted gut microbiome and almost no sleep architecture to speak of.

When we addressed these biological factors with nutrition, exercise, circadian rhythm support and practices activating her parasympathetic nervous system, her psychological symptoms improved beyond what she had achieved over several years of psychological and pharmacological therapy. The issue was more than her mind being in poor health; it was her whole system reacting to chronic biological stress.

This is the truth about emotional health, which is not some kind of anti-depression or anti-anxiety suit of armour. It is a fully-featured system that can accommodate life's challenges without getting stuck in senseless ways. The term emotional health describes a nervous system that can easily move between high and low states of activation, where thoughts and feelings align with the body's signals and where stress turns on optimising physiology rather than protective physiology.

The stress response revolution

Allow me to introduce you to your stress response system, which is perhaps the most misunderstood piece of human biology. Sapolsky's work (2017) shows that chronic stress reshapes brain circuits involved in memory, emotion and self-regulation.

I explain to my patients that our stress response is a built-in emergency system designed for life-or-death circumstances – the kind of situation where our ancestors would have encountered a predator. The instant flood of adrenaline and cortisol would have sharpened their attention and delivered a burst of energy that allowed them to react with speed and precision.

The issue today is that many of us are still operating with that ancient survival programme, though instead of a predator we face an overflowing email inbox, a demanding boss or financial pressure, all of which the primitive mind can misinterpret as threats. It is helpful to think of chronic stress as a corrupted software that interferes with the brain's operating system, making it harder to run whatever programme you want for positive change. This metaphor describes how chronic activation of a healthy system can become maladaptive in modern contexts. What was once a short-term survival mechanism has shifted into a maladaptive loop in the modern world of deadlines, bills and digital communications.

The sad irony is that the stress we accumulate while attempting to improve our lives becomes a direct obstacle to achieving those very improvements. It's exhausting to live as if danger is constant, leaving us worn down by the threats our mind manufactures automatically. There are several ways chronic stress works against transformation:

1. The prefrontal cortex becomes less active
2. Memory is impaired

3. Emotional regulation suffers
4. Physical recovery slows

1. The prefrontal cortex becomes less active

The prefrontal cortex is the part of your brain that oversees decision-making, impulse control and long-term thinking. When you're experiencing chronic stress, the prefrontal cortex becomes underactive, while the amygdala (fear centre) becomes overactive.

Imagine if your best adviser (prefrontal cortex) was always being interrupted by an overcautious security guard (amygdala), who will not let him speak. The adviser holds the strategic perspective you need, but the security guard keeps sounding alarms, making it almost impossible to plan or think clearly.

2. Memory is impaired

Prolonged stress alters the hippocampus, making it difficult to learn new behaviours or remember why you wanted to change in the first place.

This is like trying to save files onto a faulty hard drive, where the storage system has become unreliable. Useful information you just learned fails to stick or becomes distorted when you try to retrieve it.

3. Emotional regulation suffers

The neural circuits responsible for regulating your emotions become disrupted, leading to erratic mood states and reduced impulse control.

Think of your emotional thermostat malfunctioning. A small change in temperature that should barely register suddenly triggers an exaggerated response, making it difficult to maintain a stable emotional state.

4. Physical recovery slows

Stress hormones impact sleep, immune function and cellular repair, with your body becoming like a smartphone with too many apps running in the background. The battery drains more quickly, the processor overheats, and essential maintenance functions are impaired, leaving you vulnerable and depleted.

I treated a doctor named Laura, who was deep in burnout. She believed she was managing well yet could not understand why she felt so stressed. When we tested her stress hormones and found her cortisol levels to be three times higher than normal, it became clear why she experienced a heavy head, tears at the slightest trigger and a complete inability to motivate herself to do what she knew would help.

The trauma factor that most ignore

The Body Keeps the Score by Dr Bessel van der Kolk (2014) reframed trauma by showing that it does not live purely in the mind but can also leave physiological imprints altering stress responses, autonomic patterns and emotional regulation. I have found that many people unknowingly carry deep-seated, unresolved trauma that alters both mind and body by activating chronic biological stress responses, ultimately creating the very blocks they are trying to transcend.

Trauma isn't limited to soldiers in war zones or survivors of abuse. It can also include:

- Childhood emotional neglect, however unintended
- Medical procedures without adequate support
- Chronic stress with home–life instability
- Bullying or social rejection
- Accidents or injuries
- Loss of loved ones
- Financial instability

Unprocessed trauma becomes stored within the nervous system, creating patterns of hypervigilance or emotional numbness. These patterns can contribute to chronic biological stress responses. When this happens, change efforts rarely yield permanent results.

One of my patients, a high-powered executive named David, could not understand why he repeatedly sabotaged stable relationships. Together we discovered that he had been emotionally starved in childhood, which had wired his nervous system to expect abandonment. We could not begin meaningful transformation until we addressed this at the somatic level.

The science of emotional control

This might sound absurd, but in my early medical career I was shocked to realise that almost no one had been taught how to manage their own thoughts and emotions. We learn calculus in school but are supposed to know how to deal with fear, anger, sadness and stress without guidance.

Consider how strange that is. We can spend years learning algebra that most of us will never use again, but nobody teaches us what to do when our heart races before a difficult conversation, how to cope with the crushing disappointment of a setback or how to manage anxiety that keep us awake at night.

I think back to being trained as a doctor, learning the anatomy and physiology of the heart but receiving no training whatsoever on how to cope with losing a patient or supporting someone facing devastating news. I could recite the biochemical pathways of stress hormones, yet I had no idea how to manage my own stress.

You have almost certainly experienced this disparity in your own life. Perhaps you have snapped at someone you love during a hectic week and then felt overwhelming guilt, or perhaps fear around a major decision has paralysed you into indecision. Nothing is wrong with you. You were simply never taught how your emotional system works.

The neuroscience of emotional regulation

A simple way to understand the brain's emotional architecture is this: it operates on two platforms simultaneously – one fast and primitive, the other slow and sophisticated. Mastery comes from learning how these two systems interact.

As described earlier, when you experience emotions, the limbic system (your *inner alarm*, as I often call it) reacts before your conscious mind has even caught up. This ancient part of the brain evolved to detect danger instantly.

Your inner alarm sounds even before you have processed the terse email from your boss, or 'that look' your partner gave you. Like a smoke detector, your limbic system cannot distinguish between burnt toast and a real fire. It simply screams *Danger!* and floods your body with stress hormones to prepare for fight, flight or freeze.

By contrast, the prefrontal cortex, your *inner controller*, governs reasoning, planning and behavioural regulation. Crucially, though, it is much slower. By the time it arrives on the scene, your stress response has already been triggered.

Imagine walking alone down a dark street night. You hear footsteps behind you, and your inner alarm fires instantly. Adrenaline rushes through your body, your heart races, and you turn around ready to face danger, only to find an elderly man walking his tiny dog. Your inner controller eventually evaluates the scenario and calms you, but the body has already absorbed the full psychological hit.

Now imagine this same alert process happening multiple times a day, triggered not by predators but by everything from traffic to deadlines, social media notifications or even your own self-critical thoughts. It becomes easy to see why so many people feel constantly overwhelmed, despite us living in one of the safest eras in human history.

The hope: Your brain can learn new tricks

This is where things become both exciting and highly practical. Research by Davidson (2004) and Lee (2012) at the University of Wisconsin suggests that although emotional reactions occur faster than the prefrontal cortex can process, they can still be modulated into a more balanced response.

This is possible through neuroplasticity – the brain's ability to rewire itself, discussed earlier. You can train your inner controller to respond faster and more effectively, even when the inner alarm fires first. The ability to pause between a trigger and your response becomes one of the most powerful tools for reducing chronic stress and restoring vitality.

Davidson's findings are supported by more recent work. A systemic review by Calderone et al (2024) showed that mindfulness and meditation can increase cortical thickness, improve brain connectivity and reduce amygdala reactivity, all of which support stronger emotional regulation. In addition, functional neuroimaging studies have shown that mindfulness training can enhance connectivity between large-scale networks such as the default mode network (DMN), salience network (SN) and central executive network (CEN), supporting the brain's capacity to reorganise itself towards resilience.

Look at it this way: you might not be able to stop the inner alarm from reacting to perceived threats, but you can train the inner controller to engage more quickly and regulate that response more effectively. Over time, you learn to pause between trigger and your reaction, allowing the response to be calm and more measured. With practice you learn to:

- Become more aware of what is happening
- Pause long enough to assess whether the threat is real
- Choose an appropriate response rather than defaulting to instinct

It's the difference between you spending an entire morning upset about a difficult email and you taking a breath, noticing your reaction and composing a thoughtful reply. It is the difference between you snapping at your children because you are overtired and you realising the irritation is because of your workload rather than their behaviour, and adjusting before reacting.

Research in contemplative neuroscience, including work led by Dr Sara Lazar at Harvard (Lazar et al, 2005), shows that long-term meditators have greater grey-matter density in regions linked to attention, emotional regulation and self-awareness. Later longitudinal work (Hölzel et al, 2011) demonstrated that even eight weeks of mindfulness training can produce measurable structural changes in the brain. Together these findings illustrate a core principle of neuroplasticity: repeated, intentional practices gradually strengthen the neural pathways that support healthier responses.

Your body's built-in reset button

One of the simplest ways to help you regulate your emotions is something you already do thousands of times a day: breathing. Slow, deep breaths activate the parasympathetic nervous system – the body's natural calming mechanism. One of my favourite prescriptions is breathing exercises.

Research by Epel et al (2009) at UCSF shows that slow, controlled breathing lowers cortisol within minutes. A single deep breath sends your brain a clear message: *False alarm. We are safe. Stand down.*

I've seen this repeatedly in overstretched executives or anxious relatives outside hospitals, many of whom believe that smoking calms them and sharpens their concentration. That presents a fascinating paradox: how can a stimulant such as nicotine, known to raise heart rate and blood pressure, make someone feel more relaxed? The answer lies not in the cigarette but in the breathing pattern.

When smoking, people perform a slow inhale, which they briefly hold before exhaling in a long, controlled release. This mirrors the breathing techniques used in meditation and relaxation. The calming effect attributed to the cigarette is actually due to the nervous system responding to the rhythmic, controlled breathing pattern.

The tragic irony is that while activating the body's natural stress-reduction mechanisms, smokers also inhale toxins that damage their long-term health. With intentional breathwork, they could achieve the same – and often greater – relief without any of the harm.

A simple tool that changes everything

I teach patients a simple but powerful technique, which I call the STOP method – an emotional first aid kit you can use anywhere, anytime:

- **S – Stop** what you are doing. Just as you stop your car if the engine starts making a strange noise, stop your mental activity when you sense emotional intensity rising.
- **T – Take** three deep breaths. This activates your parasympathetic nervous system and gives your inner controller time to come to the scene.
- **O – Observe** your bodily sensations: tension, breath, heart rate, posture.
- **P – Proceed** with intent, making a conscious choice about your next action rather than reacting automatically.

This method works whether you are dealing with a minor irritation or major stress. My patients have used it successfully in board meetings, during arguments with their teenagers and even during medical emergencies.

The musical analogy of emotional harmony

As noted earlier, I like to think of emotions as musical notes. There are seven natural notes that can be combined in endless ways. When arranged with intention, you create a melody, a symphony or an anthem. However, when notes are thrown together randomly without thought, you end up with unbearable noise.

Similarly, we can learn to recognise our emotions and link them to experiences in a way that creates internal coherence, producing a sense of emotional harmony. In contrast, when our responses are misaligned – when a minor stressor triggers a major emotional reaction – it drains and exhausts us.

The practice of aligning your emotional responses to create harmony has lasting health benefits. Just as musicians train their ears and hands through repetition, you can through practice train your emotional circuits – a direct expression of neuroplasticity.

The gut–brain revolution

What has become one of the most thrilling areas of mental health research in recent years is our growing understanding of the gut–brain axis. The gut microbiome – the trillions of bacteria residing in your digestive system – interacts with the enteric nervous system, which contains approximately 500 million neurons and communicates with the brain extensively through the vagus nerve. Sometimes called the body's second brain, the enteric nervous system influences mood, immunity and cognition. Although the science is robust, it is still often misunderstood or oversimplified.

Perhaps even more interestingly, humans have sensed this connection for millennia. Many languages contain expressions such as *My gut feeling tells me…*, the linguistic instinct mirroring established medical knowledge.

The gut–brain connection also helps explain why targeted dietary interventions can relieve anxiety and depression in some people. Mood and cognitive performance often improve when gut health is optimised, although this is a highly individualised process requiring detailed medical evaluation and an understanding of an individual's biochemical uniqueness.

This is not about following health trends or eliminating wheat, gluten and lactose because they are unfashionable. The truth, as always, is far more complex. Some individuals might have food sensitivities or intolerances that fuel inflammation and mood dysregulation; others experience no benefit, and sometimes harm, from unnecessary restrictions. For example, if someone has a history of disordered eating they may experience fixation, accompanied by fear and anxiety related to food, when specifically eliminating foods from the diet. Others may cut out entire food groups their body needs to heal, worsening rather than improving their health.

True gut–brain work involves:

- Understanding each person's unique microbiome
- Testing for food sensitivities
- Evaluating inflammatory markers, nutrient deficiencies, medication interactions and underlying conditions

What restores balance in one person's gut–brain axis may be entirely inappropriate for another. A patient with chronic autoimmune disease may need anti-inflammatory protocols, while someone with specific genetic variants may require a completely different approach. This is why working with experienced healthcare professionals who understand the science behind gut–brain interactions is essential, and why self-diagnosis based on online advice can lead to misguided and sometimes damaging choices.

Lisa, a thirty-four-year-old teacher with chronic anxiety, had tried multiple antidepressants without improvement to her mental health. By testing her gut microbiome, we found significant bacterial imbalances. Over the course of three months, as her digestive system improved, her anxiety decreased considerably, her energy returned and she resumed yoga – something she hadn't done in seven years. She even rekindled her passion for creative writing.

Practical mental and emotional wellness

In my work with patients on mental and emotional health, we focus on building what I call *emotional fitness* – the ability to feel the full spectrum of human emotions without being dominated or derailed by them. The following schedule is designed to build emotional fitness.

SCHEDULE FOR OPTIMISING MENTAL AND EMOTIONAL WELLNESS

Daily practices

- Morning rituals that influence the rest of your day
- Physical activity that breaks down accumulated stress hormones
- Breathing exercises to activate the parasympathetic nervous system
- Evening rituals that protect and improve sleep
- Purposeful weekly chores that create structure and connection

Weekly practices

- Time in nature to reduce cortisol and stabilise mood

- Social connection with similarly growth-orientated people
- Creative expression as an outlet for emotional release
- Service to others to build purpose and perspective
- Strategic reflection and planning

Monthly practices

- Reviewing stress patterns and emotional responses
- Adjusting routines based on what genuinely supports you
- Seeking professional support when appropriate (such as therapy, coaching, medical care)
- Celebrating progress and recognising growth

Integrating body and mind

One of the most well-rounded individuals I've ever had the privilege to care for was Marcus. His collapse was no weakness but a signal from his nervous system that something needed to change. We discovered that his relentless drive was a trauma response encoded during a chaotic childhood, keeping his physiology locked in fight-or-flight mode and preventing him from experiencing the peace and satisfaction he craved.

Somatic therapy helped him to work through his child-hood trauma, and together we focused on optimising his stress-recovery systems and rebuilding genuine emotional regulation skills. Marcus not only emerged from years of depression but also regained profound creativity and joy. His business continued to thrive, now powered by love rather than fear. This illustrates a key aspect of emotional fitness: learning to shift from survival-driven patterns towards a vision led by passion and alignment. Fear alone cannot sustain transformation; only conscious alignment can.

What I would like you to take away is that mental and emotional wellbeing is not about eliminating difficult feelings or living in perpetual bliss. It is about moving through life's challenges without breaking, while preserving your ability to expand, express and enjoy.

You cannot separate mental and emotional health from physical health; together they form the foundation on which all sustainable change rests. With physical vitality, emotional steadiness and mental clarity, you can move towards your most meaningful goals from a position of power rather than fear.

Do not try to think your way out of patterns while ignoring the biology that sustains them. Treat your mental, emotional and physical health as one integrated system, and the changes you've long sought will shift from effortful to inevitable.

Take-home messages

- **Chronic stress is a major disruptor and a true barrier to change.** Persistent stress alters brain circuits, weakens emotional stability and slows physical repair. Learning stress-management techniques is essential, because only then can efforts in other areas begin to yield results.
- **The human stress system is outdated for modern life, and it needs recalibrating.** We rely on a fast inner alarm and a slower, more sophisticated inner controller. Emotional fitness comes from training the controller to take the lead so you can respond proportionately to perceived threats rather than reacting on instinct.
- **Emotional regulation is a trainable skill, not a personality trait.** Simple tools like conscious breathing or the STOP method (stop, take breaths, observe, proceed) can reset your nervous system, restore clarity and create the internal conditions in which transformation becomes possible. Like music, emotional responses create harmony when arranged intentionally and noise when thrown together chaotically.

When your nervous system is settled and your emotions integrated, your entire physiology begins to operate from safety rather than survival. A safe body does something extraordinary: it repairs, restores and regenerates. The science of longevity is built on this truth, a life lived from inner steadiness is not only happier but also healthier at a cellular level.

FIVE

Longevity: Living Better, Not Just Longer

Elizabeth, an eighty-two-year-old ex-diplomat, came to see me and delivered a truth that shifted the way I view growing old. She told me, 'I don't want to live forever, doctor. I want to soulfully live while I am still here.' This was a moment of transformation for me.

Redefining success in personal development

Elizabeth had come to see me not because she was unwell but because she wanted to make the best of what she knew would be her final years. At eighty-two she was studying Italian, plotting a Patagonia trek and working on her memoir. She also understood something that most people don't: you can add years to your life, but what really matters is adding life to your years.

This distinction is most relevant as we move into an age where a lifespan of 100 will likely become normal. The issue isn't how long you live but what kind of post-fifty, post-career decades you expect them to be: decades full of energy and life purpose, or something far less than that.

Almost every book on personal development is written as if life ends at retirement, with your twenties, thirties and forties being the peak season for achievement. What if this assumption is completely wrong, though? What if some of the best years of your life are still ahead? What if the decisions you make today determine not only how much longer you live but also how well you live?

I would like to challenge one of the greatest lies society has conditioned us to believe, that we peak at a certain age. We have been told that ageing is a straight path of decline, leading to fewer prospects, reduced vitality, shrinking opportunity. We prepare for retirement as if it is final chapter in our lives, not for what might be of the richest ones. This is not only inaccurate; it is also harmful. Once we convince ourselves that our best years are behind us, we begin to behave accordingly. We stop investing in our health because we question the point. We shy away from new experiences because we feel too old. We settle into safe patterns that slowly extinguish our spirit.

I have worked with older patients who felt better and lived with far more enthusiasm than some people thirty years younger. This had nothing to do with genetics or luck; it was understanding and application of *health span principles.*

Let's consider Margaret, who at sixty-eight had felt old and useless. Her children were grown and gone, her husband had died two years earlier, and she spent most days watching television. She moved slowly, her joints ached, and she believed this was simply what ageing felt like.

Now seventy-three years old, Margaret leads a marathon walking group and has learned conversational Spanish, and last year she launched a philanthropic project for widows, helping each to rediscover her sense of self. Now Margaret bounces into my office with stories of her latest adventures, and people assume she's in her early sixties.

What changed? Margaret now believes that ageing is not about the number of years lived but about how you live the present and the years you have left.

The longevity diet paradox

One thing that confused me when I began studying some populations with rates of exceptional longevity was that their diets were often the opposite of those recommended by modern nutritional advice.

Despite extensive use of olive oil and modest wine intake, Mediterranean communities appear healthier. The landmark PREDIMED (Prevención con Dieta Mediterránea) trial provided evidence that a Mediterranean diet supplemented with extra-virgin olive oil reduced major cardiovascular events by 30% when compared with a low-fat control diet (Estruch et al, 2018).

The Okinawans eat substantial amounts of pork, despite the widespread belief that red meat can be unhealthy. Even though the traditional French diet includes significant saturated fats, refined carbohydrates and alcohol, the French have fewer heart attacks than Americans following low-fat dietary recommendations.

Ultimately, the biggest learning is that the overall pattern of any diet matters far more than any single rule. Diet quality, social context and daily lifestyle rhythms are more important than how perfectly you adhere to dietary restrictions or macronutrient ratios.

The commonalities of blue zones include:

- Diets rich in whole, unprocessed foods
- Natural portion control practices (*hara hachi bu*)
- Communal eating
- Consistent movement throughout the day
- Stress minimisation through purpose and community

All of this underscores a crucial truth: longevity is shaped less by perfect dietary theory and far more by the biological signals your daily habits send to your cells. It is at this point – where lifestyle meets cellular mechanisms – that the science of ageing begins to take centre stage.

With this foundation in place, we can now explore what modern ageing research reveals about how the body actually grows old and, more importantly, how much of that process is within our influence.

The science of ageing: From inevitable to modifiable

Dr David Sinclair's work at Harvard Medical School (Sinclair and LaPlante, 2019) has revolutionised our understanding of ageing, which is now seen as a modifiable biological process rather than an inevitable biological destiny. Both his research and broader reviews of ageing mechanisms (eg López-Otín et al, 2013) challenge the idea that getting old must mean becoming weaker or sicker. His early research on yeast and mice showed that it is possible to extend lifespan by more than 30%, simply by activating certain cellular pathways. More recently, his work has also extended to human trials, revealing that the same longevity mechanisms operate in our own biology.

Rather than an unavoidable decline, ageing is increasingly viewed as a gradual loss of cellular information. Think of your cellular machinery as an elegantly organised library, where the instruction manuals slowly become ruined, pages fall out, and the filing system begins to fail. The remarkable scientific discovery is that this information loss can be slowed, stopped and even, in early experimental models, partially reversed, through what Sinclair refers to as *cellular reprogramming* – essentially teaching to cells to remember how to function like younger versions of themselves. Sinclair's work focuses on three foundational principles of modern longevity science:

1. **NAD+ metabolism:** NAD+ (nicotinamide adenine dinucleotide), a crucial molecule required for cellular energy and repair, becomes depleted as we age, depriving our cells of the energy required for repair (Sinclair and LaPlante, 2019). It is analogous to a vehicle that keeps running out of fuel, no matter how well the engine is maintained.

2. **Sirtuins:** These 'longevity genes' are protective proteins that defend against cellular damage. However, as we age, they become less active unless stimulated through a targeted lifestyle or metabolic signals.

3. **Cellular reprogramming:** Sinclair's research in animal models (Lu et al, 2020) demonstrates that we can, to a limited but meaningful extent, reset the biological clock within cells and train old cells how to behave as if they were young again.

What makes Sinclair's work so compelling is that many of the most effective longevity interventions do not require expensive treatments or advanced technology. The same pathways that respond to laboratory interventions in his Harvard lab react just as powerfully to specific, accessible daily habits. For example, intermittent fasting naturally boosts NAD+ and activates sirtuins, while cold exposure and specific types of exercise trigger the cellular stress responses shown to be essential for longevity.

In other words, the very signals that slow ageing at a cellular level are available to all of us, and most of them cost nothing.

Hallmarks of ageing

There are, according to scientists (López-Otín et al, 2013), nine hallmarks of ageing – the biological processes that underlie the ageing process as we know it. It helps to think of these as nine core systems that, when they begin to malfunction, can gradually shift the body from resilience to decline. Understanding the nine hallmarks of ageing helps explain why some people appear to age far more gracefully than others, regardless of chronological age.

The nine hallmarks of ageing are:

1. **Genomic instability:** Our DNA constantly accumulates damage from daily life. Think of DNA as a treasured vinyl record that accumulates scratches over time – a few scratches are acceptable, but if not polished out, they eventually add up and distort the music. In some people's DNA these scratches accumulate more rapidly, leading to greater cellular dysfunction. Fortunately, the right nutrients and lifestyle choices can help optimise cellular repair mechanisms.

2. **Telomere attrition:** Chromosomes have protective caps – telomeres – that are like the plastic tips on shoelaces. Each time a cell divides, these protective caps shorten, and when they become too short, cells can no longer function properly. Chronic psychological stress has been shown to accelerate this process, reflecting faster cellular ageing, while practices such as meditation, exercise and strong social

connections may help preserve telomere length or support the activity of telomerase, the enzyme that maintains telomeres (Epel et al, 2004).

3. **Epigenetic alterations:** DNA is like a vast instruction manual, and epigenetic markers are like bookmarks and highlighted passages that tell cells which instructions to read. As we age, these markers can shift, causing cells to read the wrong instructions at the wrong time. The good news is that those changes are potentially reversible. Unlike with DNA mutations, diet, lifestyle modifications and certain environmental factors can help reset these biological bookmarks.

4. **Loss of proteostasis:** Our cells constantly produce new proteins and clear damaged ones, acting like the quality control function in a factory. As we age, this system begins to deteriorate, allowing misfolded or damaged proteins to accumulate. These protein clumps can become toxic, contributing to neurodegenerative conditions such as Alzheimer's and Parkinson's, but certain practices like intermittent fasting and heat exposure (such as in saunas) can enhance our cells' internal cleanup systems.

5. **Deregulated nutrient-sensing:** Cells have sophisticated sensors that detect nutrients such as glucose and amino acids. These sensors

signal the cells when to grow and when to conserve resources. With age these sensors become less responsive, like a thermostat that no longer responds properly to temperature changes. This is why interventions like caloric restriction and intermittent fasting have shown promising benefits; they recalibrate the nutrient-sensing pathways, helping cells respond more appropriately to available resources.

6. **Mitochondrial dysfunction:** Mitochondria, the microscopic powerhouses inside our cells, act as little engines, generating the energy required for cellular functions. As they age, though, mitochondria become less effective, producing less energy and, in some contexts, more reactive byproducts. On the bright side, mitochondria are exquisitely sensitive to certain interventions; exercise stimulates the creation of new, more efficient mitochondria, while some key nutrients can help restore their function, allowing them to operate more as they did in youth.

7. **Cellular senescence:** Ageing cells eventually lose the ability to divide and become senescent cells, often called *zombie cells.* While still alive and metabolically active, they no longer perform their normal healthy functions. Instead, they release inflammatory compounds that damage surrounding cells, like one rotten apple spoiling the entire barrel. Research shows that the accumulation of senescent cells contributes

to chronic inflammation and age-related dysfunction, and that emerging interventions, such as senolytic and senomorphic agents, may reduce their harmful effects, although these approaches are not yet ready for routine clinical use (Saliev and Singh, 2025).

8. **Stem cell exhaustion:** Throughout the body, stem cells act as a reservoir for renewal, ready to replace damaged or dying cells. They can be considered as a biological savings account. As we age, we deplete this account, with stem cells becoming fewer in number and less capable of dividing. This explains why injuries heal more slowly as we get older. Certain factors in young blood can reactivate aged stem cells, and lifestyle interventions such as exercise and proper nutrition help preserve stem cell reserves.
9. **Altered intercellular communication:** Our cells communicate constantly, sending chemical signals to coordinate their activities. With age this communication network becomes disrupted – inflammatory signals increase while beneficial signals decrease, creating a hostile environment for healthy cells. Encouragingly, interventions such as anti-inflammatory diets and stress-reduction techniques reduce chronic inflammation, which can help restore clearer cellular communication and promote a more youthful internal environment.

I treated William, a sixty-eight-year-old engineer who came in feeling old beyond his years. Testing showed signs of accelerated ageing: shortened telomeres, raised inflammatory markers and impaired mitochondrial function. After targeted interventions directed at each hallmark – intermittent fasting, progressive exercise, stress-reduction techniques and focused nutraceutical support – within eighteen months his biological markers improved. William illustrates a central truth of modern longevity science: ageing is not fixed, and with the right inputs, it can be slowed.

Evidence-based longevity interventions

I need to make one thing clear: though scientific research has made groundbreaking advances, longevity has also been turned into a business full of hype, costly therapies and unproven claims. After examining the literature, I can say with confidence that some of the most effective interventions are among the simplest and most accessible.

Caloric restriction and intermittent fasting

Caloric restriction is one of the most powerful longevity interventions across species (Fontana, Partridge and Longo, 2010; Colman et al, 2009). Eating fewer calories while still meeting nutritional requirements activates cellular repair mechanisms (López-Lluch and Navas, 2016) and improves insulin sensitivity and inflammation profiles (Mattison et al, 2017; Longo and Mattson, 2014). Intermittent fasting offers many of these benefits without the burden of continuous calorie restriction (Harvie and Howell, 2017).

I have seen patients become more energetic and focused through intermittent fasting, which taps into an ancient biological mechanism that promotes cellular repair and resilience (de Cabo and Mattson, 2019; Longo and Panda, 2016).

Exercise: The ultimate longevity drug

If exercise were a drug, it would be the most powerful medication ever (Blair, 2009). Extensive research confirms that regular movement remains one of the most reliable predictors of long life and good health (Lee et al, 2012).

Many people mistakenly assume that strenuous workouts are superior. Extreme training can be counterproductive; the ideal goal is maintaining muscle mass, cardiovascular health and metabolic flexibility, not turning into an elite athlete.

Longevity exercise

- Cardiovascular training: 150–300 minutes of moderate activity weekly
- Strength training: Two or three sessions weekly, focusing on major muscle groups

- High-intensity intervals: One or two sessions weekly, for metabolic benefits
- Flexibility and balance: Daily movement to prevent falls and maintain mobility

I treated Robert, a seventy-two-year-old retired accountant, who thought his active days were behind him. We began with gentle walking and basic strength exercises. Two years later, he completed his first triathlon and had biomarkers better than many forty-year-olds. Robert is proof that meaningful physical rejuvenation is possible at any age.

Sleep: The foundation of longevity

Just as movement builds biological resilience during the day, sleep reinforces that resilience during the night.

Poor sleep accelerates every hallmark of ageing. Chronic sleep deprivation:

- Increases inflammation and oxidative stress
- Disrupts DNA repair mechanisms
- Disrupts hormone production
- Compromises immune function
- Accelerates cognitive decline and the deterioration of long-term brain health

Conversely, optimising sleep quality provides both immediate and long-term benefits for longevity. This is not only about duration; it is also essential to improve sleep architecture, strengthen deep sleep and support a healthy circadian rhythm.

Stress management: Protecting your telomeres

Chronic stress can shorten your telomeres. Blackburn and Epel's (2017) Nobel Prize-winning research shows that effective stress management can slow telomere shortening and, in some cases, even partially reverse it.

Importantly, stress management is not about eliminating stress, which is neither possible nor advisable. It is about developing resilience, strengthening recovery capacity and training the nervous system to return to balance rather than allowing it to remain stuck in chronic activation.

Decoding the biohacking movement: Where science ends and marketing begins

As biohacking has become popular, so too has the volume of bold claims about longevity interventions, many promoted by companies selling products for extraordinary prices. The result is a landscape where genuine science sits side by side with pure marketing, making it difficult for people to know what actually works. Allow me to help you cut through the hype.

Interventions with strong evidence

- **Cold exposure therapy.** This boosts stress tolerance and may activate pro-longevity cellular pathways (Šrámek et al, 2000; Bleakley and Davison, 2010). Cold exposure therapy is best introduced gradually to avoid potential cardiovascular risks.
- **Metformin for non-diabetics.** Early research suggests potential anti-ageing effects beyond glucose regulation (Barzilai et al, 2016). However, routine use in healthy individuals is not yet recommended without clinical supervision.
- **NAD+ supplementation.** NAD+ declines with age, impairing cellular energy and repair. Preliminary evidence indicates supplementation may support mitochondrial efficiency and DNA repair (Rajman, Chwalek and Sinclair, 2018).
- **Red light therapy.** Although still evolving, research shows promise in enhancing wound healing and cellular recovery (Avci et al, 2013).

Interventions that lack strong evidence

- Overpriced multi-ingredient supplement cocktails
- Extreme dietary protocols or juice fasts claiming 'reset' effects

- Unregulated peptide therapies
- Luxury 'longevity clinics' offering treatments with little scientific basis

The real risk isn't simply in wasting money; it's in missing the opportunity for interventions that work. I have seen patients spend tens of thousands of pounds on unproven therapies while neglecting the foundations that matter most: sleep, exercise, metabolic health, stress regulation, connection and purpose.

The truth is both reassuring and liberating: most of what extends health span is neither new nor for sale.

The blue zones solution: Secrets of the world's healthiest people

A powerful, real illustration of these principles comes from Buettner's research (2008, 2012) on the blue zones – regions where people routinely live well into their nineties and beyond without supplements, cutting-edge therapies or specialised protocols. Their exceptional longevity is driven by a handful of simple, time-tested habits (Buettner, 2017):

- Regular, natural movement built into daily life
- Solid social ties and dependable community
- A sense of purpose that goes beyond self

- Plant-forward diets with moderate portions
- Consistent sleep and stress-reduction practices
- Moderate alcohol intake, especially of red wine

What is most astonishing is how accessible these factors are. This serves as a grounding reminder: the foundations of longevity are not exotic, expensive or extreme. They are simple, sustainable and profoundly human.

Longevity and personal transformation

A knowledge of longevity fundamentally changes how we approach personal development and transformation. Instead of pursuing extreme, unsustainable changes that lead to burnout, we should focus on gentle, consistent practices that can be maintained for decades. This shift is liberating because it reminds us that growth does not need to be rushed.

Maria, a fifty-five-year-old teacher, was coping with feelings of loss following her divorce and felt that she had peaked years earlier. To her this was year one of possibly forty more years of dullness. Instead of making dramatic changes, she made small, steady adjustments, improving her health and developing new interests and friendships. Five years later, she told me those had been the happiest years of her life.

The compound effect of longevity practices

What is remarkable about longevity interventions is that their impact accumulates over time. Small, consistent practices create exponential benefits as the years go by:

- Regular physical exercise helps to maintain and build muscle mass, protecting us against frailty in later decades.
- Practising stress-management techniques supports long-term emotional stability and reduces the risk of cognitive decline.
- Social connections made today become the support system to rely on during future challenges.
- Learning new skills keeps the brain adaptable and neuroplastic, preserving mental agility throughout life.

Practical longevity protocol

This proposed schedule combines research findings with my clinical experience, offering a sustainable and practical way to promote healthy longevity at any age.

SCHEDULE FOR PROMOTING LONGEVITY

Daily practices

- Twenty to thirty minutes of physical activity
- Seven to nine hours of quality sleep

- Stress management (meditation, breathwork, time in nature)
- Social connection with people you care about
- Purposeful activity that brings meaning or fulfilment

Weekly practices

- Two or three strength training sessions
- Intermittent fasting protocol, as appropriate
- Time in nature
- Learning something new
- Service to others to reinforce purpose and perspective

Monthly practices

- Health biomarker tracking
- Social connection assessment
- Reflection on purpose, meaning and life direction
- Adjusting to routines and habits based on what is working

Annual practices

- Comprehensive health evaluation
- Goal reassessment and long-term planning
- Investment in relationship and community
- New challenges or adventures to stimulate growth

The eighty-two-year-old former diplomat I mentioned earlier, Elizabeth, embodied this philosophy. She stayed fit by walking daily and doing resistance workouts. She fed her mind by continuous learning and cultivated meaningful and supportive relationships. Most important, she met each day with curiosity and purpose.

On her last visit, she told me about the photography course she had just begun so that she could document the stories of older immigrants in her neighbourhood. That is longevity done well – not just adding years to life but adding life to years.

Whether you are in your eighties or in your teens and twenties, this work should begin now. The choices you make today shape your future. When you ground your life in the principles of healthy longevity, you don't merely extend your lifespan; you also expand the richness of your life.

We may not live forever; but we can live intelligently, vibrantly and intentionally for as long as we are here. That is the real promise of longevity.

Take-home messages

- **Ageing is malleable and far more within your influence than you have likely believed.** Modern science shows that ageing isn't a one-way decline but a set of biological processes that can be slowed, stabilised or even partially reversed. Simple, accessible habits – movement, sleep, fasting, stress regulation and nutrient-dense food – send powerful longevity signals to your cells. You're not at the mercy of your age; you're in conversation with it.

- **Focus on health span, not just lifespan – adding life to your years matters most.** The world's longest-living communities don't chase supplements, protocols or anti-ageing hacks. They move naturally, eat real food, sleep consistently, stay connected and live with purpose. Longevity isn't built on intensity but on gentle, repeated habits that keep your body resilient and your life meaningful well into later decades.
- **It's never too late to start, and small changes today compound into a radically better future.** Whether you're in your teens, thirties or eighties, every daily choice shapes your biological age. Incremental practices – strength, curiosity, stress control, connection, purposeful activity – accumulate like interest. Transformation remains possible across the entire lifespan when you follow evidence rather than hype. Your later decades can be your richest ones.

A longer life matters only if it is a richer one. The quality of your days is shaped by the silent processes constantly unfolding inside your body, and what you choose to eat is one of the greatest forces influencing them. Nutrition is not a set of rules; it is a way to help your body heal, perform and live both better and longer. In the next chapter we explore how to use food to elevate your energy, resilience and long-term health.

SIX

Identifying Your Optimal Nutrition: Science Or Sensationalism?

Anna sat across from me in my office holding a stack of diet books and on the verge of tears from sheer frustration. She had attempted a number of nutritional trends such as keto, paleo, vegan, carnivore and Mediterranean diets. They all promised to be the answer to her health concerns, but each one ultimately left her more puzzled than when she began.

'Doctor, I am so confused. I do not know what to eat anymore,' she said.

The confusion Anna was experiencing reflects the serious state of nutritional misunderstanding that I see in clinic. Even with more information available on diet and nutrition than ever before, rates of diet-related disease continue to rise.

The nutrition information paradox

This section reveals what I have discovered in my years navigating contradictory nutritional advice and working with patients in very different circumstances – from diets provided in prison canteens to those in three-star Michelin restaurants – to help you understand how your nutrition really works.

One week eggs are to blame for heart disease; the next week, they are reframed as brain-boosting superfoods. In the eighties and nineties, fat was the devil; now carbs have become vilified. This constantly changing advice can be incredibly frustrating and deeply unsettling.

When people get fed up with confusing nutrition guidance, they either become obsessed with irrelevant details or simply throw in the towel. I've watched patients swing between two destructive extremes – those obsessing about perfect eating, developing an unhealthy relationship with food; and those who say, *What's the point?* and just eat whatever, whenever. Both responses are equally damaging to health and lead people to feel overwhelmed and unable to make informed food choices.

How nutritional misinformation spreads

Nutritional confusion thrives today especially because misinformation spreads rapidly across digital platforms. A study is published suggesting blueberries may be anti-inflammatory, and within hours health bloggers are posting exaggerated claims such as 'Blueberries treat inflammation' for engagement. Nobody pays any attention to the study's limitations; the message is distorted and people everywhere hear they should eat three cups of blueberries a day. At the same time, personal trainers who possess impressive physiques but no formal nutritional education hand out, with full authority, elimination diets to anyone. Wellness coaches, some of them armed with dubious online certificates, teach people to fear entire food groups; and charismatic lifestyle gurus, with no medical or scientific training, promote protocols for conditions ranging from acne to autoimmune disease.

If a nutrition claim sounds extreme, absolute or miraculous, it is almost certainly misleading. Ask yourself three quick questions:

1. Does this claim ignore the details that actually matter?
2. Is it based on a single study rather than on a body of evidence?
3. Does someone stand to profit from your fear or enthusiasm?

If the answer to any of these is yes, be cautious.

The challenge is compounded by the fact that even fully qualified doctors often emerge from training with minimal nutritional education. In my medical training we spent just a handful of hours on nutrition – less than the time spent on obscure tropical diseases. Most of my colleagues can prescribe diabetes medication, but few can explain why a patient may be better off having protein with each meal.

This gap is systemic: medical curricula focus on treating disease rather than preventing it. We learn to diagnose nutrient deficiencies after they have caused advanced complications, but we are rarely taught how to prevent them. The result? Doctors are brilliant at managing disease but poorly equipped to teach effective nutrition.

Nutrition schools have similar issues. Most programmes remain rooted in outdated nutritional models such as the old fat-is-harmful theory, simplistic calorie counting that ignores hormonal and metabolic context, and one-size-fits-all rules that overlook individual variability. I still meet registered dietitians who believe all calories are equal and that meal timing doesn't matter. They continue teaching principles preserved in outdated textbooks, which do not reflect modern science on circadian rhythms, gut microbiome diversity and nutrient–gene interactions.

The foundation: Understanding your biochemistry

Before considering any dietary strategy, it's important to understand how your body metabolises nutrients. After years of reviewing much research and treating patients with every imaginable dietary preference, I've observed several principles that promote health and longevity. This is not textbook biology; it's the practical knowledge that will help you make informed dietary decisions rather than following the latest dietary trend.

Macronutrients and micronutrients: What your body actually uses

Proteins, fats and carbohydrates are not interchangeable; each supports distinct biological roles:

- **Protein** – provides amino acids essential for tissue repair, immune function and hormone production
- **Fat** – supports hormone synthesis, brain health and the absorption of fat-soluble vitamins
- **Carbohydrates** – supply rapid energy and support physical performance

Vitamins and minerals act as essential biochemical cofactors. When they are lacking, key reactions slow down or stall, creating metabolic bottlenecks. Because modern agriculture and food processing lower nutrient density, micronutrient deficiencies have become more common in some populations.

Individual variation: Why no single diet works for everyone

Your nutritional needs are determined by your genetics, gut microbiome composition, stress levels, activity patterns and current health. These factors direct how you metabolise nutrients, which foods you tolerate and which metabolites your gut bacteria produce as a result.

This is why no single dietary pattern – whether Mediterranean, ketogenic, vegan or others – applies universally.

Nutrient density and anti-inflammatory eating

Nutrient-dense foods rich in vitamins, minerals, fibre and phytonutrients protect long-term health and help reduce chronic inflammation. Seafood, offal, legumes, nuts, seeds, whole grains, and colourful fruits and vegetables offer the greatest nutritional return per calorie.

Since, as discussed earlier, chronic inflammation accelerates ageing, foods that reduce inflammation are particularly valuable. These include:

- Omega-3 fatty acids
- Polyphenol-rich berries, tea and cocoa

- Herbs and spices such as turmeric and ginger
- Dietary fibre, which nourishes beneficial gut bacteria

Please believe me: no single food is a miracle; it's consistent patterns that matter.

The myth of superfoods

The wellness industry has convinced many people that exotic ingredients offer unique, transformative benefits. In reality, açaí berries are no more 'super' than blueberries, and quinoa is no more exceptional than other whole grains. What changes health is habitual dietary quality, not rare imports.

I treated Patricia, a health-conscious woman spending hundreds each month on imported berries, powders and supplements while skipping meals, sleeping poorly and ignoring chronic stress. Once we focused on simple fundamentals – regular meals with adequate protein, together with whole foods, hydration, stress management and restorative sleep – her energy improved dramatically. The basics, not superfoods, are what delivered the change.

Whole foods over processed foods

Among all nutritional advice, this is one of the principles most consistently supported by scientific evidence.

Ultra-processed foods are strongly associated with chronic disease and reduced lifespan (Monteiro et al, 2019). In a study of more than 100,000 adults, every 10% increase in ultra-processed food intake was linked to a 14% rise in all-cause mortality (Rico-Campà et al, 2019), a finding echoed across multiple large cohorts (Srour et al, 2019).

Long-lived populations provide a practical illustration of these findings. The world's healthiest communities – such as those studied in the blue zones – eat diets composed mainly of whole, minimally processed foods prepared in simple, traditional ways (Buettner and Skemp, 2016; Buettner, 2012; Willcox, Willcox and Suzuki, 2007). They do not follow complex nutritional rules; they eat food that looks close to how it was when grown and harvested.

The conclusion is clear: prioritising whole foods over processed alternatives is one of the most reliable and impactful strategies for long-term health and longevity.

Protein: The most underrated nutrient

Protein is still the most overlooked cornerstone of good health. It supports muscle maintenance, immune function, wound healing, hormone and enzyme production, and metabolic regulation, yet many people live with a degree of protein insufficiency, often without realising it. Subtle signs include constant hunger, slow recovery, feeling weaker with age or, despite exercising, struggling to build muscle.

After around the age of forty, the natural decline in muscle mass (sarcopenia) begins to accelerate, but this is largely preventable with adequate protein and regular resistance training. Protein also helps keep appetite in check by triggering satiety signals such as GLP-1 (glucagon-like peptide-1) and PYY (peptide YY). This is the same pathway mimicked by medications like semaglutide (Ozempic) and tirzepatide (Mounjaro), which explains their powerful appetite-suppressing effects. However, the downside is clear: when appetite drops too far, people often eat insufficient protein and lose muscle. These medications work best when paired with sufficient protein, not as a substitute for it.

Protein and fasting: Finding what works for you

Protein and fasting are often presented as competing philosophies, but in reality they are simply different tools. The 'best' approach depends entirely on your age, goals and physiology.

If you are older, recovering from training or trying to build or maintain strength, spreading your protein across two or three meals usually serves you best. If you are younger, metabolically healthy or prioritising longevity and metabolic flexibility, time-restricted eating or one to two protein-rich meals per day can work extremely well.

The essential point is simple: many people do not consume enough protein, no matter how many meals they eat.

Fasting can complement protein intake rather than contradict it, and when used wisely, it activates some of the most powerful repair mechanisms we know of.

The science of fasting

Fasting is one of the most misunderstood and yet most powerful nutritional tools we have. It is not a trend. It is a biological rhythm our bodies evolved with, and modern science is finally catching up with what our ancestors practised intuitively.

When food is paused for a meaningful period (usually twelve to sixteen hours or more), the body shifts into a deeper form of maintenance and repair. These changes touch almost every system.

Below are the key mechanisms – explained simply, supported by research and rooted in real clinical experience:

1. Autophagy – your cells' housekeeping system
2. Metabolic switching
3. Natural growth hormone release

4. Reduced inflammation
5. Brain benefits – neuroplasticity and clarity

1. Autophagy – your cells' housekeeping system

One of the most profound things fasting triggers is autophagy – your body's way of clearing damaged proteins, old organelles and cellular debris. Fasting simply gives your cells the space to clean, repair and rebuild.

The scientific understanding of autophagy marked a revolutionary breakthrough, earning Yoshinori Ohsumi the 2016 Nobel Prize for identifying the genes that control it (Ohsumi, 2014; Mizushima et al, 2008).

Autophagy naturally declines with age. Studies show that interventions that extend lifespan often do so by stimulating this internal recycling system (Rubinsztein, Mariño and Kroemer, 2011).

2. Metabolic switching

After twelve to twenty-four hours without food, you transition from burning glucose to burning fat.

Your liver produces ketones, a highly efficient fuel that supports both energy and mental clarity. This ability is called *metabolic flexibility*, and most of us have lost it due to constant eating, grazing and snacking, yet our ancestors relied on this switch for survival.

Regaining metabolic flexibility improves insulin sensitivity, stabilises energy and enhances metabolic health.

3. Natural growth hormone release

Fasting increases growth hormone release significantly, sometimes severalfold in certain contexts.

This matters because growth hormone protects lean muscle, supports tissue repair, improves sleep architecture and assists in fat metabolism.

People often try to mimic these benefits with injections. Synthetic hormones come with risks, though (water retention, joint pain, glucose dysregulation), and they lack the elegant hormonal orchestration that fasting provides naturally.

4. Reduced inflammation

Earlier in the book I explained how chronic inflammation accelerates biological ageing. Fasting can lower inflammatory cytokines such as TNF-α and IL-6 (Johnson et al, 2007; Aksungar, Topkaya and Akyildiz, 2007) in some contexts.

It also activates the AMPK pathway, a master regulator of energy balance that influences metabolic and anti-inflammatory pathways (Mattson, Longo and Harvie, 2017; Longo and Mattson, 2014).

This is why many people report less joint stiffness, improved digestion and clearer thinking during fasting.

5. Brain benefits – neuroplasticity and clarity

Extended fasting increases BDNF (brain-derived neurotrophic factor), which supports the growth of new neurons and the strengthening of neural circuits (Mattson et al, 2018).

Many patients report feeling unusually focused or motivated while fasting. Far from being just a psychological perception, these effects are driven by measurable changes in the brain.

Fasting protocols that work

Drawing on both scientific evidence and clinical practice, four fasting approaches stand out as the most practical, effective and sustainable:

1. 16:8 time-restricted eating

This is a gentle, highly practical entry point in which eating is confined to an eight-hour window and fasting spans the remaining sixteen. Most people find this routine easy to adopt and maintain because it works with rather than against the body's natural rhythms.

What I see most often in clinic is that this rhythm steadies appetite, reduces the desire for late-night grazing and supports more stable energy through the day. It's flexible enough to fit into almost any schedule, and when paired with balanced meals, it becomes one of the simplest ways to support metabolic health without feeling like a diet.

2. One meal a day (OMAD)

OMAD is a more intensive approach that provides extended periods of autophagy and ketosis. Many patients choose it for the mental clarity it *may* provide and for its simplicity, though the single daily meal must be nutrient-dense, especially in protein. OMAD is not suitable for everyone. If you have medical conditions or take medication, you should consult your doctor before considering this approach.

3. Intermittent fasting (5:2)

With five days of normal eating and two days of reduced intake (around 500–600 kcal per day), this pattern echoes the natural cycles of scarcity and abundance our bodies evolved with, and many people find it surprisingly sustainable. The two lighter days give the digestive system a rest, support insulin sensitivity and may help stabilise appetite across the week.

Clinically, I see this approach work particularly well for people with metabolic concerns who struggle with daily fasting windows. The structure is clear, the rhythm is predictable, and the routine doesn't interfere too much with family meals or social eating. When nourishing, protein-rich meals are included on both fasting and non-fasting days, this approach can provide a gentle but powerful reset for the body.

4. Occasional, supervised 24–72-hour fasts

These fasts can deepen the adaptive benefits. Any fast beyond twenty-four hours should ideally be medically supervised, and fasting beyond seventy-two hours always requires strict supervision.

When patients follow one of these fasting patterns consistently, I repeatedly observe the same shifts in clinical practice: improvements in insulin resistance, reductions in blood pressure, and the kind of mental clarity many describe as 'feeling switched on again'. One patient, a forty-nine-year-old paramedic, put it simply: 'I didn't feel restricted. I felt lighter, in my body and in my mind.' That is the power of metabolic switching.

Fasting safety and considerations

Before going any further, let me make one thing clear: fasting is not appropriate for everyone. For example, if you have a history of eating disorders, are pregnant or breastfeeding, have certain medical conditions or take medications that require food, fasting should be avoided. Speak with a doctor who understands your medical history.

For most healthy adults, however, gradually introducing fasting is both safe and beneficial. Many people find it helpful to begin with a twelve-hour overnight fast and, as their bodies adapt, extend it to fourteen or sixteen. This gentle progression helps prevent the fatigue, headaches and irritability people experience when they jump in too aggressively.

Finding your individual mix

The more we study human biology, the more we realise how differently each of us processes, absorbs and responds to food. Your optimal way of eating depends on several intertwined factors:

1. **Genetics:** Subtle variations in genes influence how you metabolise caffeine, break down carbohydrates and respond to fats.
2. **Gut microbiome:** Your trillions-strong bacterial community plays a major role in digestion, inflammation and blood-sugar regulation, which explains why a high-fibre diet feels wonderful for some and disastrous for others.
3. **Metabolic state:** Insulin sensitivity, metabolic flexibility and current health status all shape what foods you thrive on.

4. **Activity level:** The nutritional requirements of an athlete, for example, differ dramatically from those of a sedentary person.
5. **Lifestyle and cultural preferences:** Any diet that ignores your routines, family life, culture or access to food is doomed to fail, regardless of how perfect it looks on paper.

I once treated identical twin sisters, who were genetically indistinguishable and raised in the same environment, yet their bodies thrived on completely different eating patterns. One responded beautifully to a Mediterranean-style approach; the other felt and performed far better on a diet higher in protein and fats with fewer carbohydrates. Their microbiomes, stress levels, activity patterns and metabolic markers were nothing alike.

This is why, for example, some people feel renewed on OMAD while others function far better with two or three meals. Your biology, not popular rules or trends, is what ultimately guides the right approach.

Practical nutritional guidelines

People differ widely, so no single eating pattern suits everyone. Across all this variation, though, a few principles consistently support almost every body:

- Prioritising whole foods, when possible choosing minimally processed options

- Favouring fresh and seasonal foods (and using frozen vegetables when needed, as they retain nutrients well)
- Ensuring sufficient protein, typically around 1–1.2 grams per kilogram of body weight daily, with older adults or highly active individuals possibly benefiting from slightly higher amounts
- Loading your plate with vegetables – ideally, half the plate at most meals
- Staying hydrated, with pale yellow urine being your best guide
- Practising portion awareness, eating until satisfied rather than stuffed (with satiety signals taking about twenty minutes to register)
- Allowing flexibility, following the eighty-twenty rule – eating well most of the time but making space for social meals and cultural food experiences

Rather than strict rules, these principles create a steady framework – the kind of gentle structure that both your body and your psychology can thrive in.

If applying all of them feels like too much, start smaller, focusing on the three habits with the highest biological return on investment:

1. Eating enough protein – the single strongest protector of muscle, metabolism and healthy ageing

2. Limiting ultra-processed foods – where even a reduction of 20–30% can improve blood sugar, inflammation and energy levels
3. Maintaining an eating window that lets your body rest – with twelve to fourteen hours' overnight fasting being enough to support repair without feeling restrictive

If you do nothing else, these three habits alone are likely to improve almost every relevant metabolic marker.

Integrating nutrition into real life

Anna, whom I introduced earlier in this chapter, beautifully illustrates the concept of integrating nutrition into real life. Instead of attempting to prescribe a 'perfect diet', we focused on habits she could maintain. She adopted a simple, real-food Mediterranean-style pattern, combined with intermittent fasting and supported by a few targeted supplements to correct deficiencies. Importantly, she also allowed herself the flexibility to enjoy meals with friends and family without guilt. Within six months her energy stabilised, her sleep improved and she permanently shed the twenty pounds she had unsuccessfully tried to lose for years. More importantly, she felt confident making food choices on her own.

That is what I want for you – not another restrictive plan that collapses under real life but a sustainable way of eating that supports your health, honours your culture and fits the life you want to live. Nutrition is one the pillars of health, working in concert with sleep, exercise, stress management and meaningful relationships. Striving for dietary perfection while neglecting these other foundations simply doesn't work.

Your goal is not to find the perfect diet. It is to build a way of eating that fuels your body, supports your identity and sustains the life you want to lead.

Ultimately, nutrition is not a performance to perfect but a relationship to cultivate. It is the daily dialogue between your biology and your choices – the quiet habit that either builds your future health or erodes it. You do not need exotic foods, rigid rules or online approval. What you need is clarity, consistency and a way of eating that strengthens your efforts to grow into a healthier, steadier version of yourself. When you start listening to your body and feeding it with intention rather than impulse or fear, something remarkable happens: your energy rises, your mind steadies, and the real you begins to emerge.

Take-home messages

- **Nutrition confusion is common, and scientific evidence brings clarity.** Behind the noise, the strongest science remains remarkably consistent: whole, minimally processed foods protect long-term health, adequate protein maintains muscle and metabolism, and nutrient density lowers inflammation and supports cellular repair. These patterns are supported across large epidemiological studies, metabolic research and the dietary habits of the world's longest-living populations.

- **Fasting is simple but biologically powerful.** Intermittent fasting isn't a trend. It triggers mechanisms recognised in modern longevity science, including autophagy, metabolic switching, increased growth hormone and reduced proinflammatory cytokines. These shifts enhance cellular resilience, insulin sensitivity and brain plasticity. Used appropriately, fasting is one of the most scientifically grounded tools for metabolic and cellular health.
- **Personalised nutrition reflects how biology truly works.** One size cannot fit all. Genetics, microbiome composition, metabolic flexibility and lifestyle patterns all influence how individuals respond to the same foods. Studies repeatedly show striking differences in blood-sugar responses and nutrient metabolism between people eating identical meals. This is why the 'perfect diet' doesn't exist, but personalised, flexible principles can align eating with your biology for lasting health.

Food fuels your cells, but relationships fuel your nervous system. You can learn to eat perfectly and still be biologically inflamed, emotionally dysregulated or chronically stressed if you are disconnected or lonely. Human connection is one of the most potent health interventions we have, and in the next chapter I reveal why.

SEVEN

Relationships: The Social Prescription

My phone rang at 2am. A heart attack had struck George, an eighty-nine-year-old former CEO I was working with. I headed to the hospital, thinking he would be surrounded by family and friends. Instead, I found him alone.

George had built a business empire, growing wealthy and well connected – a man of achievement in every ego-driven way that society measures success. However, his impressive sports and academic achievements did not matter as he faced his own mortality lying alone in a hospital bed. Connection is what counted, and George had little.

'Doc,' he whispered, 'I have it all – everything I ever thought I wanted – except a real person to share it with.'

Reflecting on George, I am reminded that his life exemplifies what has been documented over eighty years in the 'Harvard Study of Adult Development' (Harvard Second Generation Study, ongoing). In their book, *The Good Life*, the study's leaders, Waldinger and Schulz (2023), emphasise that good relationships are the key to a happier and healthier life. This critical component, however, remains strangely overlooked in most approaches to personal transformation.

George's words transported me back to a defining time in my life. I was at a crossroads, torn between the security of my career in finance and the calling I felt towards medicine. To help clarify which path to follow, I volunteered at Trinity Hospice in London, spending time with patients who were terminally ill. Something that struck deeply there was realising that when people know they are dying, they speak with brutal honesty.

What I heard repeatedly was not regret for what they had done but anguish over what they had failed to do. Some regretted mistakes, of course, but the deepest, most painful regrets centred on opportunities they had let slip away out of fear. They spoke of powerful attractions to others that they had not dared to act on, opinions they hadn't felt courageous enough to voice, potential life-changing experiences they had never pursued. Guilt and the fear of judgement had kept them from being their authentic selves. They had played safe, conformed to expectations and avoided discomfort. Now that they were facing death, that very caution left them feeling profoundly incomplete.

As I listened further, a deeper pattern became clear. Those people's regrets were not only about missed careers or unexpressed opinions in isolation. At the heart of almost every lament was a feeling of failure to connect authentically, not pursuing relationships that mattered, not being honest with loved ones, not finding their true community. They had spent their lives conforming, fitting in with the wrong groups, pretending to be someone they weren't. The real tragedy wasn't physical loneliness; it was living a life fundamentally alienated from who they truly were.

This experience at Trinity Hospice made me understand what a healthy life truly means. You can follow every health recommendation, but without real connections life is likely to remain hollow. The most peaceful passings were among those who had loved and been loved in return.

As I listened to the regrets of chances not taken, something crystallised in me. I didn't want to reach the end of my life wondering *What if?* That clarity pushed me to leave my secure path and pursue a career in medicine.

The medical case for relationships

A fact that surprises many people is that social isolation is as damaging to your health as well-established behavioural risks factors, often compared to the effects of smoking fifteen cigarettes a day. Decades of rigorous epidemiological research confirms this. One major study of 308,849 participants (Holt-Lunstad, Smith and Layton, 2010) found that people with strong social relationships have a 50% greater likelihood of survival than those who are socially isolated.

Modern science now explains why and how high-quality relationships influence key physiological systems:

1. **Immune response:** People with strong social connections mount more robust immune responses. In a landmark study, Cohen et al (1997) exposed 276 volunteers to rhinovirus; those with diverse social networks were significantly less likely to develop cold symptoms. Later, Cole et al (2007) demonstrated why: loneliness alters gene expression, increasing inflammatory activity while suppressing antiviral defences.
2. **Stress buffering:** Social support dampens the body's stress response. Eisenberger et al (2011) showed via functional MRI scans that even

holding a loved one's hand during a stressful task reduces activity in the brain's threat-detection regions and activated reward circuits.

3. **Cardiovascular health:** Relationship quality predicts heart health. Research by the Framingham Heart Study (Eaker et al, 2007) showed that being happily partnered was more protective for cardiovascular health than good cholesterol levels or blood pressure.
4. **Cognitive resilience:** Social engagement protects the ageing brain. Findings from the Rush Memory and Ageing Project (Bennett et al, 2006) revealed that each increase in social network score reduced Alzheimer's risk by 41%.
5. **Pain management:** Meaningful connections modulate pain perception. Master et al (2009) found that simply looking at a picture of a loved one during a painful stimulus was associated with a reduction in subjective pain ratings and decreased activity in neural pain circuits.

I have seen these effects repeatedly in practice. Patients with meaningful relationships recover faster after surgery, adhere better to treatment and maintain healthier routines over time. Most importantly, they retain hope. Relationships generate a positive feedback loop: connection strengthens health, and improved health deepens connection.

The biology of connection

Humans evolved as social creatures, and our biology still reflects this truth. When we connect meaningfully with others, the body releases oxytocin – the *bonding hormone* – which can quietly influence cardiovascular, stress-response and immune pathways, including effects on blood pressure, cortisol regulation and aspects of healing. Far from being only a feel-good chemical, oxytocin alters physiology in ways similar to therapeutic medications, reducing blood pressure and heart rate, lowering cortisol, strengthening immune function, enhancing healing and improving insulin sensitivity, and it may even influence pain tolerance.

I saw this clearly in Maria, a fifty-two-year-old teacher, who was recovering from a painful divorce. Her blood pressure was elevated, her sleep was disrupted, and her spirit was flat. I encouraged her to reach out to old friends and join a writing group. Three months later, without medication, Maria's blood pressure had normalised and her mood had lifted considerably. Social connection healed what medication alone could not.

Quality over quantity: What research shows

The most important lesson from relationship research is simple, and – as noted earlier in this chapter – it's the quality of your relationships rather than the quantity that determines their impact on your health. You can have hundreds of online connections and still feel profoundly alone, while just a few close, supportive relationships can transform your wellbeing.

Anthropologist Robin Dunbar (1992) showed that while humans can maintain around 150 meaningful social connections, only a small circle – usually a small group of three to five people – provides the depth of support that truly matters.

This reinforced something I had already begun to see. Through my early career in law, finance and even medicine, I had been surrounded by colleagues and acquaintances yet had very few genuine friendships. I was constantly focused on others but had neglected my own relational needs. It wasn't until my own transformation that I understood that deep friendship is not a luxury for personal happiness; it is essential for survival.

Family relationships: The first blueprint

Our earliest relationships leave a significant imprint on our health. Research on adverse childhood experiences shows that early relationship trauma carries physical and psychological consequences well into adulthood (Felitti et al, 1998; Anda et al, 2006). The hopeful part is this: thanks to neuroplasticity, healthy relationships formed later in life can repair much of that early damage (Rutter, 2012).

I have seen this many times. When I worked as a doctor in a prison, I discovered that one of my patients, former gang member David, had never experienced a safe and supportive relationship. Through therapy and group work he learned to trust and relate to others. Watching him build his first healthy connections in his thirties was a powerful reminder that our relationship patterns are not fixed; they can be rewired at any age.

The friendship prescription

Friendships in adulthood don't form automatically; you have to cultivate them. Unlike in childhood, when friendships grow out of proximity, adult life demands intention. It's no wonder so many struggle – modern cities, long work hours and digital communication make real connection harder.

The encouraging news is that research consistently shows what strengthens friendships:

- **Regular contact.** Small, repeated gestures matter far more than grand efforts. Research by Jeffrey Hall (2018) suggests it takes roughly 200 hours to form a close friendship, and that our efforts are most effective when spread over time rather than in intense bursts.
- **Shared activities.** When people move, laugh or focus together, their brain activity

synchronises – a form of behavioural synchrony that deepens connection – whether, for example, through exercises, hobbies, volunteering or simply shared meals.

- **Mutual support.** Healthy friendships aren't one-sided; there is a natural rhythm of giving and receiving.
- **Emotional openness.** Vulnerability – sharing fears, dreams, struggles and joys – is what upgrades a friendship from pleasant to meaningful.
- **Reliability.** Being reliable is the glue that holds a friendship together.

I saw this transformation in Sandra, a forty-five-year-old executive who felt successful everywhere except in her personal life. Together we built a realistic 'friendship prescription'. She joined a book club, tried rock climbing and gently deepened existing acquaintanceships. Within a year she had formed two authentic friendships that reshaped her emotional landscape.

Marriage and partnership: The health benefits

Falling in love is one of the most extraordinary human experiences. It is almost magical – that time when you observe someone in a crowded environment and suddenly experience an indescribably strong connection.

Neuroscience shows that intense romantic attraction can activate the brain's reward system within milliseconds – faster than almost any other stimulus. When it comes to health, though, it isn't the spark that matters most; more important is the quality of the relationship that follows.

Strong, supportive partnerships consistently predict better health outcomes, while poor-quality relationships can be damaging. Observational and longitudinal studies show that people in troubled marriages exhibit higher levels of inflammatory markers, such as interleukin-6 and C-reactive protein, along with declines in cellular immune function, compared with those in higher-quality relationships (Kiecolt-Glaser et al, 2006; Robles et al, 2014). Hostile or unsupportive interactions have also been linked to slower wound healing and weakened immune responses, illustrating the physiological consequences of relational stress (Holt-Lunstad, Smith and Layton et al, 2010).

Healthy partnerships tend to share some core traits:

- **Conflict as growth.** Conflict is inevitable; what matters is how it's handled. Avoiding criticism, contempt, defensiveness and stonewalling keeps disagreements constructive rather than destructive.
- **Shared meaning.** Common values, a sense of purpose and aligned vision for the future create emotional coherence and long-term stability.

- **Physical affection.** Touch and intimacy release oxytocin, laying the neurological foundation for trust and bonding.
- **Independence within interdependence.** The healthiest couples maintain individuality while building something bigger. It is about two strong selves choosing connection, not losing oneself in the other.

I've seen both sides of this equation in practice.

I remember Lisa, an energetic thirty-eight-year-old artist who suffered with chronic headaches, anxiety and insomnia – all symptoms that deepened over years in a marriage overshadowed by constant criticism. Her body was reacting to emotional attrition.

Conversely, I watched something remarkable unfold with John and Mary, who had been married for twenty-five years. They came to me feeling depressed and with chronic health issues. With the couples therapy and communication work I encouraged, they rediscovered the connection that had once anchored their marriage. As their relationship healed, so did their health.

Loneliness

We live in a time when you can reach almost anyone, anywhere, at any time, and yet people feel more disconnected than ever. Young adults may have thousands of online followers, but many report feeling lonelier than elderly residents in care homes. Something fundamental has gone wrong in how we connect.

Digital communication can of course be helpful. It bridges distance, allows communities to be formed on shared interests and can sustain relationships that might otherwise fade. It cannot, though, replace the deep biological and psychological nourishment that comes from physically sharing space with another human being.

Research reflects the paradox. In a study of nearly 1,800 young adults, those who used social media the most were also the loneliest (Primack et al, 2017). Another study following more than 5,000 people found that face-to-face interactions predicted later happiness and health, while digital interactions predicted the opposite (Shakya and Christakis, 2017).

Connection is not the same as contact.

The loneliness epidemic

Loneliness has become a global public-health crisis. The World Health Organization's Commission on Social Connection recently described loneliness and social isolation as a serious health threat, affecting nearly one in six people worldwide (WHO, 2025a). Chronic social isolation has also been linked to a roughly 50% increased risk of developing dementia (Holt-Lunstad et al, 2015). The physiological and psychological toll of isolation is profound, with loneliness contributing to premature mortality and serious health consequences comparable to other recognised risk factors such as smoking or obesity (WHO, 2025b).

Several forces are driving this epidemic:

- Families scattered across continents
- Work cultures that prioritise productivity over people
- Urban living that erodes community
- A digital world that distracts us with constant contact while depriving us of genuine connection

Human beings are wired for presence, not perpetual scrolling.

Why presence matters

Face-to-face interaction triggers profound biological responses that no device can replicate. In-person conversation dramatically increases oxytocin, the bonding hormone that supports trust, healing, emotional safety and pain tolerance. Phone calls produce modest increases; texting and social media produce almost none (Seltzer, Ziegler and Pollak, 2010).

We also experience 'embodied synchrony', where our breathing, heart rhythms and subtle brain patterns fall into a kind of partnership with those around us. This is an ancient biological language that can only be activated in person. This is why you cannot text your way into feeling seen, held or understood; your nervous system knows the difference.

None of this means that technology is essentially harmful. Used wisely, it can enhance connection. For example, during the pandemic, video calls kept families emotionally close and allowed support groups to continue their life-saving work. Technology bridged distances that would otherwise have been devastating.

The magic happens when we use digital tools as bridges to real connection – a WhatsApp group that leads to a walk in the park, a dating app that leads to a real relationship, a fitness tracker that motivates friends to train together – rather than as replacements for it.

Trouble arises when the bridge becomes the destination – when a text replaces a voice, when emojis replace emotion, when online likes become a substitute for love. Screens can coordinate connection, but they cannot create the neurobiology of connection. True relationships happen in the flesh.

The social skills that build connection

The good news is that strong relationships are not reserved only for people who are naturally sociable.

Social abilities are learnable, practicable and transformative skills. They don't just improve your relationships; they also shape how your body regulates stress, immunity and emotional stability. Learnable social skills include:

- **Active listening.** The most powerful relational skill you can learn is genuine listening – giving someone your full attention without planning your response. Listening is a physiological gift because it signals safety to another person's nervous system.

  When people feel heard, their stress hormones drop immediately (Reis and Shaver, 1988). Brain scans show that when two people truly connect, their brain patterns begin to mirror each other – a process known as neural coupling (Stephens, Silbert and Hasson, 2010).

- **Empathy.** Empathy is not sentimentality; it is a biological bridge between nervous systems. In a study of patients with the common cold (Rakel et al, 2011), those who experienced high clinician empathy mounted double the immune response of those who received standard care. Their bodies healed faster.

  Being understood is medicine – not metaphorically but biologically.

- **Boundaries and authentic communication.** Boundaries are often misunderstood as signs of selfishness, but research shows the opposite. People who constantly suppress their needs or avoid conflict to preserve relationships experience poorer health outcomes. Healthy boundaries and honest communication create mutual respect and deepen trust.

- **Healing through practice.** I once worked with Robert, a forty-five-year-old engineer paralysed by social anxiety. Through simple training in social skills and gradual exposure to real-world interactions, his life changed within months. His insomnia resolved, his blood pressure normalised, and he told me he felt like he had 'finally re-entered life'.

  Relationships are not just emotional experiences; they are biological events.

- **Cultivating community.** Community, whether through faith, hobbies, volunteering or local networks, is one of the strongest predictors of resilience. People embedded in community heal more quickly, live longer and face adversity with greater strength.

  Community is not a luxury; it is a survival mechanism.

The ripple effect of relationships

George, the man whose heart attack opened this chapter, is one of the clearest examples of the ripple effect of relationships. For the first time in decades he reached out to old friends, joined a men's group at his church and volunteered at a literacy programme. The transformation was remarkable. His blood pressure dropped, his sleep improved and his energy returned. The real shift, though, was internal – he felt reconnected to life itself.

Relationships give back what you invest. They are virtuous cycles of meaning, support and renewal.

Take-home messages

- **Connection is medicine; isolation is a health risk.** Decades of research show that strong relationships protect health as powerfully as exercise, nourishing food and good sleep. Social isolation, on the other hand, raises mortality risk as much as smoking. Meaningful connection lowers inflammation, strengthens immunity, buffers stress and supports cardiovascular and cognitive health. Relationships are not optional; they are fundamentally essential for biological health.
- **The quality of relationships reshapes your biology.** A few close, supportive relationships provide most of the emotional and physiological benefits. High-quality bonds calm the threat response, regulate cortisol, improve recovery and build resilience across the lifespan. From early

childhood to late adulthood, healthy relationships can repair psychological wounds and support neuroplastic change.

- **Connection is built, not found.** Learnable social skills like active listening, empathy, clear boundaries and honest communication measurably improve health by lowering stress, enhancing immune responses and deepening emotional safety. Though digital contact can be useful, it cannot replace the biological impact of face-to-face presence. Strong relationships grow through consistent attention, shared activities and intentional investment.

Healthy relationships stabilise the nervous system, and love transforms it. Loving relationships can trigger beneficial changes in hormones, reduce inflammation, strengthen immunity and even slow cellular ageing. The power of love is not soft or sentimental; it is biologically profound, deserving an entire chapter of its own.

EIGHT

Love: The Neuroscience Of Connection

During a consultation, a question stopped me in my tracks: 'Doctor, can love heal?'

Catherine was forty-three, newly divorced, and for the last two years had been living inside what she called a grey fog. No medication had lifted her symptoms of depression. She woke each morning exhausted, and each evening she collapsed into bed. This persisted until she met James, a gentle veterinarian who made her laugh for the first time in years.

After seeing him a couple of times, she said, 'I know this sounds ridiculous, but I feel different. Not just emotionally, but physically. I've got energy. I'm sleeping.

Yesterday I walked willingly. Is falling in love healing me?'

She thought she was imagining things. She wasn't. Many patients describe similar patterns – a sudden return of energy, clarity and calm – long before their blood tests change.

Love is medicine

The effects of love are not mystical; they are measurable shifts in hormones, neural circuits and inflammatory pathways that modern tools can now observe in real time. What Catherine was experiencing was not a fantasy or coincidence. It was biology – powerful, measurable and increasingly understood through modern science.

Across continents and cultures, evidence converges on one truth: love heals.

People who experience deep social connections live longer than their counterparts (Holt-Lunstad, Smith and Layton, 2010). Social participation across midlife is associated with up to 50% lower risk of dementia (Sommerlad et al, 2023).

A vast meta-analysis of 148 studies involving over 300,000 participants arrived at a conclusion more striking than any pharmaceutical trial. Strong, loving relationships were associated with a 50% increase in likelihood of survival – an effect comparable to factors such as quitting smoking, exercising regularly or maintaining healthy weight (Holt-Lunstad, Smith and Layton, 2010).

This is not just about longer life. It is about richer, steadier, more meaningful life.

Healing traditions across the world recognised this long before modern science. Traditional Chinese medicine links emotional harmony to physical wellbeing. The ancient Indian system of medicine, Ayurveda, teaches that love strengthens *ojas* – the body's deepest source of resilience. Indigenous cultures have long understood that individual healing is inseparable from communal support and love, and science is only now beginning to catch up.

The neurobiology of love

When Catherine described how she felt when meeting James – the ease, the warmth, the inexplicable lift – she was describing a neurochemical event. Brain-imaging studies show that early romantic attraction activates reward and attention circuits rapidly and intensely (Fisher et al, 2016).

This surge releases dopamine, norepinephrine and phenylethylamine in varying degrees, sharpening attention, heightening motivation and increasing energy. The story does not end at euphoria, though.

Love can support beneficial neural rewiring. When people experience secure love, research shows that brain activity shifts in ways that calm fear circuits, reduce stress and strengthen reward and regulation networks (Acevedo et al, 2012).

Early-stage romantic love has been shown to lower cortisol, soothing the nervous system (Weisman et al, 2014). The release of bonding hormones such as oxytocin and vasopressin deepens attachment and may influence sleep quality, stress regulation and immune pathways in ways that support overall physiological balance (Kiecolt-Glaser and Wilson, 2017).

Love is also associated with changes in immune markers. People who feel more loving and compassionate show lower inflammatory cytokines and stronger antiviral responses (Stellar et al, 2015). Even telomeres – those protective caps that shrink under chronic stress – tend to be longer in people who feel securely supported, most likely because lower stress indirectly supports healthier cellular ageing rather than love directly altering telomere biology (Epel et al, 2004; Blackburn and Epel, 2012). Love is not metaphorically medicinal; it functions almost like molecular medicine.

Love and the heart

Love does not only lift mood; it reaches the cardiovascular system with astonishing speed. Simple, loving touch – holding hands, hugging, a gentle arm around the shoulders – is associated with measurable reductions in blood pressure and heart rate, while also increasing heart rate variability, one of the strongest indicators of cardiovascular resilience (Holt-Lunstad, Birmingham and Jones, 2008).

By contrast, large population studies (American Heart Association, 2023) show that chronic loneliness is associated with a 29% higher risk of heart attack and cardiovascular death.

The heart is not just a pump. It is a profoundly social organ, shaped by our connections.

Love and the mind

Catherine's transformation was not only emotional; it reflected deep physiological change within the brain.

Loving relationships provide what neuroscientists call co-regulation – the ability of one person's nervous system to steady another. This is why a calm partner can soothe anxiety far more effectively than any technique practised alone.

Neuroimaging work by Lewis, Amini and Lannon (2000) shows that healthy attachment strengthens the prefrontal cortex, the brain region responsible for emotional regulation, clarity of decision-making and stress management, while reducing activity in fear-based circuits.

Love, in essence, gives the brain a safer operating environment.

Different loves, different medicines

Love is not one thing. It arrives in many forms, each activating distinct biological pathways:

- **Romantic love.** Intense, energising and biologically potent, romantic love activates reward circuits strongly, producing effects that can feel similar to those of mood elevation medications.
- **Companionate love.** This is the deeper, steadier affection that grows in long-term relationships. It produces the most sustained benefits – lower inflammation, stronger immunity and greater emotional stability.
- **Friendship love.** Love shared in friendships is reliable, nourishing and quietly life-extending. Close friends act as 'chosen family', buffering stress without the volatility that sometimes accompanies romantic relationships.

- **Love for pets.** Even brief interactions with pets raise oxytocin, lower blood pressure and increase immune markers. Petting a dog for just eighteen minutes was associated with increased IgA (immunoglobulin A) levels in college students (Katch, 2022).

Love comes in many forms, all of which have medicinal properties.

Six months after our first conversation, Catherine returned to clinic looking like a different person. Her depression scores had dropped from severe to minimal. Her fatigue had resolved completely. Her sleep had normalised, and even her inflammatory and stress-related blood markers had improved. These are all changes that previous medications had not produced.

What struck me most was her voice which was lighter, clearer, full of life. 'I feel alive again, and not just because James is wonderful. Loving him reminded me how to love everyone else – my friends, my family...even myself.'

Love had not simply elevated her mood. It had recalibrated her physiology, expanded her relationships and reignited her sense of purpose. In addition to healing Catherine, love restored her to herself.

The architecture of love

Our capacity to experience love and its health benefits is shaped by a number of factors throughout life.

Attachment styles

Everyone's primary attachment style is formed early in life, with four main categories:

1. **Secure attachment** – makes intimacy natural and stabilises the nervous system, supporting longevity and immunity
2. **Anxious attachment** – heightens vigilance, increasing stress and undermining love's health benefits
3. **Avoidant attachment** – protects against vulnerability but restricts access to connection and its physiological rewards
4. **Disorganised attachment** – often rooted in trauma, creates a painful push–pull relationship with intimacy

An attachment style does not need to be one's destiny, though, as the brain can rewire at any age.

I have seen patients shift from anxious to secure, avoidant to open, fearful to trusting, all through steady, consistent experiences of healthy connection.

Love across the lifespan

The expression of love changes over time, but its biological importance does not. In young adulthood, love shapes identity, resilience and stress-buffering ability. In midlife, love stabilises us during the years of greatest responsibility and strain. In later life, love becomes the primary source of cognitive protection, emotional wellbeing and meaning.

At every age, love is protective.

Cultivating love as medicine

Our ability to express and enjoy love is not purely down to luck. It can always be learned, practised and strengthened.

Science identifies several practices that reliably expand our capacity for love:

1. **Self-compassion** – is shown to reduce inflammation and increase resilience (Neff, 2003)
2. **Gratitude** – strengthens neural pathways for connection
3. **Loving-kindness meditation** – increases positive emotion and structural brain changes linked to empathy
4. **Acts of service** – activates reward pathways for both giver and receiver

5. **Physical touch** – releases oxytocin and lowers stress
6. **Deep listening** – synchronises neural activity and builds authentic intimacy

These practices are not sentimental. They are physiological upgrades.

Love as a catalyst for transformation

Perhaps the most extraordinary aspect of love is that it does not merely heal illness; it also accelerates transformation. When we feel genuinely loved and accepted, fear decreases and courage expands. We become willing to change, to risk something new, to grow.

David, a corporate lawyer battling addiction, began his recovery with a single letter from his teenage daughter telling him she loved him regardless of his mistakes and believed he could change. That unconditional acceptance became his anchor.

Sarah, a high-achieving executive imprisoned by perfectionism, achieved transformation only when she allowed herself to be seen – not flawless, but real. Love gave her permission to drop the armour.

Love is not soft; it is transformative. It addresses the most beneficial and life-changing aspects covered in this book – including sleep, nutrition, movement, stress, relationships – and makes them achievable.

Love: The bridge to becoming

By now, a pattern is clear. Everything in this book – the neuroscience, the biology, the clinical evidence – forms the architecture of transformation.

Love is the bridge to becoming because it:

- Stabilises the nervous system
- Rewires the brain
- Expands emotional courage
- Deepens relationships
- Enhances meaning
- Accelerates behavioural change

Love turns knowledge into embodiment. Love turns intention into action. Love turns survival into becoming.

Catherine discovered this. Many of my patients have discovered this. Now, so will you.

Where love leads

Catherine once asked me if love could heal, but she discovered something greater. Love not only heals the wounds of who we have been; it also opens the doorway to who we are capable of growing into next.

That brings us to the question at the heart of this book: how do you create a new self? Love places you on the bridge. The next chapter shows you how to cross it.

Take-home messages

- **Love is biological, and its effects are measurable.** Love isn't poetic exaggeration; it produces concrete physiological change. Secure, supportive love lowers cortisol, reduces inflammation, strengthens immunity and may even influence cellular ageing. Touch, affection and emotional safety trigger oxytocin and parasympathetic calming, improving cardiovascular health, sleep and resilience. Love is not metaphorical medicine; it functions similarly to molecular medicine.
- **Different forms of love support health, each in unique ways.** Romantic love activates reward circuits and boosts motivation; companionate love stabilises mood, reduces inflammation and strengthens long-term wellbeing; deep friendships act as protective buffers against stress. Even loving interactions with pets raise oxytocin and soften the stress response. Love comes in many forms, and each delivers its own biological benefit.
- **Love reshapes the brain, and resilience can be learned.** Healthy connection strengthens the prefrontal cortex, quiets fear circuits and

> creates co-regulation, where one person's calm nervous system steadies another. These changes enhance emotional clarity and stress tolerance. Crucially, the skills that cultivate love – self-compassion, gratitude, touch, acts of service and deep listening – are all trainable behaviours that activate the same neural pathways. Love is a daily practice, not an accident.

Love can accelerate the reshaping of both your biology and your identity. It creates a depth of safety that allows you to take risks, grow and experience yourself more fully. Transformation is never dependent on falling in love, but when it happens, a romantic connection can act as a catalyst, helping to initiate, enhance or accelerate the journey of becoming. It adds an extra layer of enrichment to the alignment of your biology, your emotions and your deeper self.

NINE
Creating The New You: Evidence-Based Transformation

The man sitting across from me, Thomas, had changed. Two years earlier, he had been a 280-pound powerful corporate executive, battling diabetes and depression while heading towards a divorce. He felt he had been living someone else's life, trapped in routines that gave him neither joy nor purpose. Now he weighed 180 pounds, exercised regularly, had reconciled with his wife and had set up a non-profit organisation supporting underprivileged children.

It wasn't Thomas's physical transformation that struck me most. It was the clarity in his gaze, the quiet confidence of a man who had finally come home to himself.

'Doctor,' he said, 'I feel like I slept for twenty years and just woke up.'

This transformation is a reminder of something profound: our circumstances, our habits, even our identity, are more malleable than we imagine. As highlighted repeatedly throughout the book, real change requires far more than willpower. It requires an understanding of the biological, psychological and relational forces that shape human behaviour.

This chapter brings everything together. It shows how all the systems we've explored – your body, your mind, your relationships, your environment – interact to create lasting, meaningful transformation.

Integration: A whole-person approach

The ideas in this book are not separate elements to be improved one at a time. They form a single, living system, and sustainable change happens only when that system shifts as a whole.

You cannot optimise nutrition while neglecting your relationships.

You cannot chase ambitious goals while running on chronic sleep loss.

You cannot strive for psychological growth while ignoring the biological foundations that support it.

Thomas's transformation happened for this very reason. He didn't 'fix' one area of his life. He redesigned the whole system in alignment with the person he wanted to become. It wasn't a diet. It wasn't a fitness plan. It was complete, coherent recalibration.

Integration is where real change begins and where it finally holds.

The neuroscience of change

For decades the prevailing belief was that the adult brain was largely hard-wired – that personality, habits and capability were largely set by early adulthood. As touched on earlier in the book, modern neuroscience has dismantled that myth, and this concept deserves deeper attention here.

Neuroplasticity, the lifelong capacity of the brain to reorganise itself, varies across regions but remains an active process. Your brain keeps reshaping itself through what you practise, what you focus on and the emotional patterns you return to, gradually forming the internal architecture that supports who you are growing into. The old belief that people become too old to change is not based on science; it is a misunderstanding. Research demonstrates that the brain continuously remodels itself through focused, repeated, meaningful experiences (Merzenich, Van Vleet and Nahum, 2014).

When I first studied philosophy, Heraclitus's axiom *panta rhei* (everything flows) struck me as poetic rather than scientific. Years later I realised how precisely it describes human change. Nothing in us is static. We are always in movement, always in some stage of becoming.

Every time you practise a new skill, sit with discomfort, interrupt an old pattern or choose a different response, your brain is being rewired. Change feels difficult at first because the pathways are still forming, but it becomes easier as those pathways strengthen and your new way of being becomes familiar.

Transformation isn't based on magic or luck. It's about the biology that allows you to become the person you've always known you could be.

Focused attention: The neuroplasticity switch

Neuroplasticity accelerates when actions are paired with focused attention. Research, including work by Bavelier (Bavelier et al, 2012), shows that states of sustained, deliberate attention enhance the brain's capacity to learn by strengthening the neural pathways associated with the new behaviour. Focused engagement increases the release of neurotransmitters such as acetylcholine and norepinephrine, the brain's natural 'learning amplifiers' that consolidate these changes.

I saw this vividly with Mario, a fifty-two-year-old senior executive trapped in cycles of anxiety and catastrophic thinking. Instead of loosely trying to be more mindful, he committed to three daily twenty-minute sessions of focused mindfulness. After six weeks, his anxiety had halved. His mind felt clearer and more grounded, and his emotional reactivity had softened.

Focused attention drives real change. Whatever you repeatedly bring into awareness becomes the structure your mind quietly starts to build on.

The Goldilocks zone of growth

Significant brain change happens within what psychologists call the *zone of proximal development*, where challenges stretch you but don't overwhelm you.

Woollett and Maguire's (2011) study of London taxi drivers showed that significant hippocampal changes occurred only when their training reached its most challenging stages. Early, easier phases of practice produced no measurable structural change, and tasks that were overwhelmingly difficult also did not lead to gains. Woollett and Maguire's findings highlight a key principle of neuroplasticity: the brain tends to adapt most effectively within the 'Goldilocks zone', when challenges are demanding but still achievable. Growth is generally supported by progressive challenge.

Sarah, a forty-five-year-old teacher terrified of public speaking, repeatedly threw herself into high-stakes presentations, each time freezing. Her brain was overwhelmed. We shifted her into the Goldilocks zone via a series of steps:

1. Recording herself privately
2. Speaking to one trusted friend
3. Speaking to a small group
4. Presenting to a classroom

Within weeks her confidence soared. Her brain had been given the space to adapt.

Repetition + consistency = habit

Neural pathways strengthen through repetition, and neurons that fire together tend to wire together (Hebb, 1949).

Regular practice is the biological foundation of habit. This explains why crash diets fail but gradual shifts succeed, why weekend warriors get injured while daily movers stay resilient, why cramming produces short-term recall but not long-term mastery.

Lasting change is achieved not by intensity but through consistency.

Emotion: The memory-enhancing system

Emotionally meaningful experiences are encoded more strongly as memories than purely intellectual ones. This is because the amygdala–hippocampus–prefrontal network, a key circuit influencing emotionally enhanced memory, becomes more active when information carries emotional significance – particularly when change resonates with personal values (McGaugh, 2004).

Rebecca, for example, intellectually understood every cognitive technique for overcoming depression, but nothing shifted until she connected with her deepest value: being emotionally present for her teenage daughter. That emotional clarity activated motivation circuits that logic alone never reached.

Transformation must touch the heart as well as the mind.

Rest and regroup: The quiet engine of change

Sleep isn't downtime. It's one of the most active, restorative processes your body has. During sleep your brain strengthens learning, repairs tissue, balances hormones and lays down the neural pathways that make change possible.

Most people misunderstand sleep entirely. We expect ourselves to leap from full alertness into deep rest, as if a mind racing at a hundred miles an hour could simply switch off on command. It can't. Your nervous system needs a bridge.

In clinic I often explain the importance of sleep hygiene not as a rigid set of rules but as practical ways of preparing the body and mind for rest. Getting high-quality sleep is something you can achieve through simple, repeatable practices like:

- Dimming lights an hour before bed
- Shutting down blue-light devices
- Establishing a predictable routine
- Engaging in calming activities

Elena, a marketing director living on four hours' sleep per night, resisted at first because she believed rest was indulgent. Once she adopted a nightly routine, her productivity soared. Her mood stabilised, her relationships deepened, and her presence returned.

Sleep doesn't change your life on its own, but it gives you the foundation that makes every other part of transformation easier.

The power of silence: Meditation science

As a lawyer turned doctor, I once regarded meditation as a pleasant distraction, but learning to meditate in a monastery in Thailand changed that. I realised meditation was not about escaping thought or relaxing; it was about relating differently to thought.

Meditation is now one of the most studied mental-health practices in neuroscience, and it is also one of my favourite prescriptions.

As mentioned in Chapter Four, Dr Sara Lazar's research at Harvard first showed that experienced meditators exhibit increased grey-matter density in regions involved in attention and emotional regulation (Lazar et al, 2005). Subsequent studies, including those by Hölzel et al (2011), reported similar structural changes following mindfulness-based programmes. Together, this work reinforces a broader truth about transformation: when healthier responses are practised consistently, the brain adapts, gradually wiring these patterns into pathways that become increasingly automatic.

What fascinated me most was how quickly these changes can begin. Just eight weeks of practice is enough to produce measurable alterations in the brain. It's a reminder that the brain responds generously to even small, steady commitments.

Meditation is also associated with reduced amygdala reactivity, the overactive smoke detector of the mind. People that mediate consistently describe the same lived experience: the emergence of a 'pause button' – a moment's space between stress and reaction where choice becomes possible.

Justin, a hedge-fund manager sceptical of meditation, began with five minutes a day after his second panic attack. Months later, his team described him as calmer, wiser, more deliberate. He described himself as 'finally able to breathe'.

The best part is that meditation requires no equipment, no complexity; it requires only presence. Benefits include:

- Reduced stress and cortisol
- Strengthened immunity
- Improved sleep
- Reduced pain sensitivity
- Enhanced attention and executive function

Types of meditation

Meditation is far simpler than the modern world makes it. Apps or meditation classes can be helpful when you're starting out, as they can give you structure and help you understand the basics, but real meditation is ultimately practised in silence and without external guidance. It's in the quiet that the mind learns to settle and where the deeper changes take root. The core forms include:

1. **Mindfulness meditation:** Observing thoughts, sensations and feelings without judgement, returning gently to the present
2. **Loving-kindness meditation:** Cultivating compassion for yourself, loved ones, neutral people, difficult people and ultimately all beings
3. **Concentration meditation:** Focusing on a single anchor such as the breath or a mantra
4. **Body-scan meditation:** Observing physical sensations with interest and acceptance
5. **Movement meditation:** Practising mindful walking, yoga or tai chi – especially helpful for those who struggle with stillness

Even brief practice makes a measurable difference. One study (Tang et al, 2007) found that just twenty minutes a day for five days improved emotional regulation and attention. It's a powerful reminder that you don't need long sessions or perfect technique. What matters most is showing up consistently.

Beyond meditation: Other transformative practices

Transformation thrives when the body, mind and environment are aligned. Some of the most potent, accessible tools include:

- **Journalling and self-reflection.** Writing helps organise emotion, clarify values, identify patterns and process difficult experiences. Research by Pennebaker (1997) shows expressive writing can improve immune function and reduce psychological distress.
- **Nature exposure and forest bathing.** Spending time in nature is associated with lowered stress hormones, enhanced immunity, improved mood and restored cognitive function. In Japan, *shinrin-yoku* – forest bathing – is simply the act of immersing yourself in nature, using all your senses.
- **Creative expression and flow states.** Creativity supports transformation through problem solving, emotional release, self-belief and states of profound absorption (or flow). Recent research (Rosen et al, 2024; Jean-Berluche, 2024) suggests that creative engagement is associated with improvements in cognitive, emotional and social wellbeing, although these studies describe correlations rather than direct causal effects.

- **Service and contribution.** Helping others can trigger a 'helper's high' – a physiological uplift driven by neurochemicals such as dopamine, endorphins and oxytocin. People who volunteer tend to have lower rates of depression and longer lifespans (Jenkinson et al, 2013).

True service requires presence. This raises an important question: why do the very people dedicated to helping and healing others – doctors – experience such high rates of stress and burnout? A major reason is that modern, time-pressured medical systems restrict genuine connection. Service heals when it is relational, human and unhurried.

The change process: A medical model

Transformation rarely happens in a straight line. In practice it unfolds in stages – a progression I've seen in many patients:

- **Stage 1: Preparation and assessment**
  - Assess your life domains honestly
  - Clarify where change is needed
  - Identify underlying health issues
  - Establish support and accountability
  - Set realistic timelines

- **Stage 2: Implementation and practice**
  - Begin with small, sustainable changes
  - Seek consistency, not perfection
  - Track progress with meaningful metrics
  - Modify changes based on feedback
  - Expect an adjustment phase
- **Stage 3: Integration and habit building**
  - Expand changes gradually
  - Learn from setbacks
  - Create maintenance strategies
  - Shape your environment to support the new behaviour
  - Develop adaptability
- **Stage 4: Transformation**
  - New behaviours feel natural
  - Identity shifts to support them
  - Challenges become opportunities
  - Growth becomes self-reinforcing

Understanding this pattern of change helps you recognise where you are, what comes next and why the process sometimes feels uneven. It gives you a sense of direction rather than perfection, and the guidance you need to keep moving forward. When you understand these stages, change stops feeling mysterious. The process becomes something you can work with – one step, one adjustment, one choice at a time – until the person you're becoming no longer feels distant but inevitable.

Common obstacles and evidence-based solutions

Every meaningful change encounters resistance. In this process the resistance comes not from lack of willpower but from the natural tension between biology, emotions and environment. These forces can slow progress, confuse your expectations or make the path feel harder than it should. None of this signals failure; it simply highlights where the system needs support. The obstacles most commonly arise in three main areas, listed here with evidence-based ways to move through them with clarity and momentum:

1. **Biological challenges –** Chronic stress, poor sleep, nutrient deficiencies, hormonal dysregulation, inflammation

   Solutions: Optimisation of sleep, nutrition, exercise and stress management, with medical support when needed

2. **Psychological barriers –** Limiting beliefs, perfectionism, unclear values, low motivation, fear of change

   Solutions: Meditation, journalling, therapy,

value clarification and structured support systems.

3. **Social restraints** – Unsupportive relationships, family pressures, lack of community, isolation, toxic social comparison

   Solutions: Communicating your goals, building supportive networks, seeking professional guidance when needed

Professional support

Seeking help is wisdom, not a weakness, and experts can accelerate transformation and spare you years of unnecessary struggle. They help you clear blind spots, steady the process and build skills that are difficult to develop alone. Professionals that can provide that support include:

- Medical professionals to optimise biological foundations
- Therapists to help you process trauma and build emotional regulation
- Coaches and mentors to guide skill development
- Support groups to provide community and shared experience

Measuring progress: A data-driven transformation

Tracking your progress accurately gives you an honest picture and helps prevent discouragement, protecting you from the tricks your emotions can play on you. Measuring progress lets you see the truth of your efforts, even on days when your mind tells a different story. Measurements are possible in three main areas:

1. **Biological metrics** – Body composition, inflammatory markers, sleep quality, HRV (heart rate variability) and stress biomarkers, energy and cognition performance measures
2. **Psychological metrics** – Mood and anxiety scores, coping effectiveness, life satisfaction, goal achievement, self-efficacy
3. **Social metrics** – Relationship quality, community engagement, communication patterns, support availability, sense of belonging

Progress becomes undeniable when it's visible. Once you can see it, you naturally align more closely with the person you are evolving into.

Sustainability: The long game

For change to last, it needs the right foundations – the inner conditions that make transformation not just possible but also sustainable. Lasting change grows from steadiness, not strain – from steps you can keep taking in your daily life rather than measures you need to struggle to maintain.

Lasting transformation requires:

- **Alignment with your nature** – respecting biology and temperament
- **Intrinsic motivation** – with changes that feel meaningful
- **Adaptability** – with the flexibility to refine your approach
- **Self-compassion** – understanding setbacks without collapse
- **Integration** – replacing old habits with habits that nourish you

Your personal transformation protocol

Drawing together all the principles above, I've outlined a simple protocol you can tailor to yourself – a framework to guide your next steps with clarity and confidence.

PERSONAL TRANSFORMATION SCHEDULE

Month 1: Foundation assessment

- Comprehensive health assessment
- Review relationships and support
- Clarify values and motivations
- Identify obstacles and resources

Months 2–4: Building the foundations

- Optimise sleep, nutrition, exercise and stress
- Address medical issues
- Begin mindfulness practice
- Strengthen supportive relationships

Months 5–8: Skill development

- Build core skills for your goals
- Emotional regulation and communication
- Test new behaviours in low-risk settings

Months 9–12: Integration and expansion

- Increase challenge and complexity
- Integrate new behaviours across settings
- Develop long-term maintenance strategies
- Begin supporting others

Second year and beyond: Mastery and service

- Refine your transformation toolkit
- Serve others on similar journeys
- Pursue new growth opportunities
- Align with a cause that reflects your values

Use this as a guide, not a rulebook. Shape it to your life, adjust it as you grow, and let it support your evolution into a steadier, truer version of yourself.

The compound effect of transformation

When biology, psychology and environment align, small changes accumulate into sweeping transformation.

Thomas, the patient mentioned at the beginning of this chapter, illustrates this compound effect beautifully. Exercise improved his sleep. Better sleep improved his emotional steadiness, which in turn helped to heal his marriage. Healing his marriage reduced stress, creating space for a renewed sense of purpose, and that sense of purpose eventually led him to serve others.

Upward trajectories are real. Transformation compounds.

Becoming who you truly are

Transformation does not turn you into someone else. It reveals the person life's noise has obscured.

The science is clear: you can change at any age and far more profoundly than once imagined. The only remaining question is the one only you can answer: *will you continue living a life shaped by your past conditioning, or will you consciously create the life that, deep down, you know is yours to live?*

Take-home messages

- **Transformation is possible because you are biologically built to evolve.** You are biologically built to evolve at any age and in any chapter of life. Neuroplasticity shows that your brain never stops adapting. Every choice you make sends a signal that can strengthen your biology. You are not confined by who you've been; you are shaped by what you do next. You are not stuck; you are unfinished.
- **Lasting change is simple, and small actions create remarkable outcomes.** The most profound transformations don't come from heroic intensity but from steady, repeated practices that accumulate over time. Each night of good sleep, each nourishing choice, each moment of calm attention is a step towards the person you are growing into, and your biology strengthens every small choice.
- **Alignment creates inevitability, and coherence turns effort into momentum.** When all parts of your life move in the same direction, change becomes inevitable. As shown throughout this book and supported by medical science, aligning your body, mind, relationships and values doesn't

just make change easier; it unlocks the version of you that has been waiting underneath. This is the moment change stops being a struggle and begins to feel like your new reality.

Transformation is not mysterious or magic; it is the product of aligned biology and intention, emotion aligned with purpose, and identity aligned with truth. When these systems work together, change stops being a battle and becomes a trajectory.

Conclusion: Your Journey Begins Now

As I pen these last lines, I am humbled by the extraordinary improvements I've witnessed in many patients, including inmates who have found purpose, city professionals whose frenzied pace has been calmed, elderly patients for whom the twilight years of life are now invigorated. All have taught me about the boundless capacity for human transformation.

Let me be absolutely clear about what sets *The Science of Becoming* apart. True transformation – becoming who you truly are – isn't something you can force with positive thinking or motivational mantras alone. It begins with understanding yourself more deeply, in recognising that your body is a complex biological system with its own rhythms, needs and intelligence. When you learn to work with your body's processes rather than against them, change stops feeling like a battle and starts becoming something that unfolds naturally.

I've seen diabetic patients for whom positive thinking alone won't persuade their pancreas to make more insulin, but who discover that optimal stress management supports blood-sugar regulation. Patients with chronic pain finding that focusing on sleep, a low-inflammation diet and adequate stress response can, alongside medical care, provide significant relief. Depressed individuals for whom improving health gut and optimising exercise and circadian rhythms has taken them further than therapy and medication combined.

The journey you are about to embark on will be both the most difficult and the most rewarding work you will ever undertake. It takes courage to see how your lifestyle may be causing health problems and to accept your limitations honestly. It takes wisdom to work with your biology rather than fight it. It takes persistence and patience – above all, patience – to allow changes to unfold at their own pace. Feed your biology what it needs – food, sleep, movement, stress managing techniques and emotional connections – and it will become a powerful ally.

What I really wish you to be certain about is that becoming you is not only possible; it is your birthright. Right now, you have within you everything you need to begin the process of change and grow into the person you have always sensed you could or should be. The science is clear, the path is outlined, and the tools required are available. Your transformation can begin today, in this moment, with the next choice you make. Make it count.

Perfection isn't required. You don't have to have all the answers, and you do not have to transform yourself overnight. You simply need to begin, taking one step at a time, with compassion for yourself and understanding what your body can do naturally, and simply trust the process.

When you provide the right conditions, your biology will support your aspirations. When you invest in your relationships with purpose and consistency, they will flourish. Your transformation is not only about improving your own life; it is about growing into the kind of person who contributes to making the world a little brighter.

The science of becoming is the art of unleashing the person you truly are underneath all the conditioning, fears and limitations accumulated over the years. Remember, you are not broken and you do not need fixing. You are a human being capable of extraordinary growth once you unfold your full potential.

The door is open. It is time to begin.

> 'The best time to plant a tree was twenty years ago.
> The second-best time is now.'
> — Chinese proverb

Dr J Crespo

References

Acevedo, BP et al (2012) 'Neural Correlates of Long-Term Intense Romantic Love', *Social Cognitive and Affective Neuroscience*, 7/2, 145–159, https://doi.org/10.1093/scan/nsq092

Aksungar, FB, Topkaya, AE and Akyildiz, M (2007) 'Interleukin-6, C-Reactive Protein and Biochemical Parameters During Prolonged Intermittent Fasting', *Annals of Nutrition and Metabolism*, 51/1, 88–95, https://doi.org/10.1159/000100954

American Heart Association (2023) 'Social Isolation and Loneliness Increase the Risk of Death from Heart Attack, Stroke', *AHA/ASA Newsroom*, https://newsroom.heart.org/news/social-isolation-and-loneliness-increase-the-risk-of-death-from-heart-attack-stroke, accessed 29 September 2025

Anda, RF et al (2006) 'The Enduring Effects of Abuse and Related Adverse Experiences in Childhood', *European Archives of Psychiatry and Clinical*

Neuroscience, 256/3, 174–186, https://doi.org/10.1007/s00406-005-0624-4

Avci, P et al (2013) 'Low-Level Laser (Light) Therapy (LLLT) in Skin: Stimulating, healing, restoring', *Seminars in Cutaneous Medicine and Surgery*, 32/1, 41–52, https://pubmed.ncbi.nlm.nih.gov/24049929, accessed 28 September 2025

Barzilai, N et al (2016) 'Metformin as a Tool to Target Aging', *Cell Metabolism*, 23/6, 1060–1065, https://doi.org/10.1016/j.cmet.2016.05.011

Bavelier, D et al (2012) 'Brain Plasticity Through the Life Span: Learning to learn and action video games', *Annual Review of Neuroscience*, 35, 391–416, https://doi.org/10.1146/annurev-neuro-060909-152832

Bennett, DA et al (2006) 'The Effect of Social Networks on the Relation Between Alzheimer's Disease Pathology and Level of Cognitive Function in Old People: A longitudinal cohort study', *The Lancet Neurology*, 5/5, 406–412, https://doi.org/10.1016/s1474-4422(06)70417-3

Bernad, BC et al (2024) 'Epigenetic and Coping Mechanisms of Stress in Affective Disorders: A scoping review', *Medicina*, 60/5, 709, https://doi.org/10.3390/medicina60050709

Blackburn, EH and Epel, ES (2012) 'Telomeres and Adversity: Too toxic to ignore', *Nature*, 490/7419, 169–171, https://doi.org/10.1038/490169a

Blackburn, EH and Epel, ES (2017) *The Telomere Effect: A revolutionary approach to living younger, healthier, longer*, Grand Central Publishing

Blair, SN (2009) 'Physical Inactivity: The biggest public health problem of the 21st century', *British Journal of Sports Medicine*, 43/1, 1–2, https://bjsm.bmj.com/content/43/1/1, accessed 27 September 2025

Bleakley, CM and Davison, GW (2010) 'What Is the Biochemical and Physiological Rationale for Using Cold-Water Immersion in Sports Recovery? A systematic review', *British Journal of Sports Medicine*, 44/3, 179–187, https://doi.org/10.1136/bjsm.2009.065565

Bower, JE and Kuhlman, KR (2023) 'Psychoneuroimmunology: An introduction to immune-to-brain communication and its implications for clinical psychology', *Annual Review of Clinical Psychology*, 19, 331–359, https://doi.org/10.1146/annurev-clinpsy-080621-045153

Buettner, D (2008) *The Blue Zones: Lessons for living longer from the people who've lived the longest*, National Geographic

Buettner, D (2012) *The Blue Zones: 9 lessons for living longer from the people who've lived the longest*, 2nd ed, National Geographic Books

Buettner, D (2017) *The Blue Zones of Happiness: Lessons from the world's happiest people*, National Geographic Books

Buettner, D and Skemp, S (2016) 'Blue Zones: Lessons from the world's longest lived', *American Journal of Lifestyle Medicine*, 10/5, 318–321, https://doi.org/10.1177/1559827616637066

Calderone, A et al (2024) 'Neurobiological Changes Induced by Mindfulness and Meditation: A systematic review', *Biomedicines*, 12/11, 2613, https://doi.org/10.3390/biomedicines12112613

Clear, J (2018) *Atomic Habits: An easy and proven way to build good habits and break bad ones*, Avery

Cohen, O (2003) 'Endotoxin-induced changes in human working and declarative memory associate with cleavage of plasma "readthrough" acetylcholinesterase', *Journal of Molecular Neuroscience*, 21/3, 199–212, https://doi.org/10.1385/JMN:21:3:199

Cohen, S et al (1997) 'Social Ties and Susceptibility to the Common Cold', *JAMA*, 277/24, 1940–1944, https://pubmed.ncbi.nlm.nih.gov/9200634, accessed 28 September 2025

Cole, SW et al (2007) 'Social Regulation of Gene Expression in Human Leukocytes', *Genome Biology*, 8/9, R189, https://doi.org/10.1186/gb-2007-8-9-r189

Colman, RJ et al (2009) 'Caloric Restriction Delays Disease Onset and Mortality in Rhesus Monkeys', *Science*, 325/5937, 201–204, https://doi.org/10.1126/science.1173635

Covey, SR (1989) *The 7 Habits of Highly Effective People: Restoring the character ethic*, Free Press

Damasio, A (1994) *Descartes' Error: Emotion, reason, and the human brain*, GP Putnam's Sons

Damasio, A (2010) *Self Comes to Mind: Constructing the conscious brain*, Pantheon Books

Dantzer, R (2009) 'Cytokine, Sickness Behavior, and Depression', *Immunology and Allergy Clinics of North America*, 29/2, 247–264, https://doi.org/10.1016/j.iac.2009.02.002

Davidson, RJ (2004) 'Well-Being and Affective Style: Neural substrates and biobehavioural correlates', *Philosophical Transactions of the Royal Society B*, 359/1449, 1395–1411, https://doi.org/10.1098/rstb.2004.1510

Davidson, RJ (2012) ''Well-being and affective style: neural substrates and biobehavioral correlates',

Philosophical Transactions of the Royal Society B: Biological Sciences, 359/1449, 1395–1411, https://doi.org/10.1098/rstb.2004.1510

de Cabo, R and Mattson, MP (2019) 'Effects of Intermittent Fasting on Health, Aging, and Disease', *New England Journal of Medicine*, 381/26, 2541–2551, https://doi.org/10.1056/nejmra1905136

Doidge, N (2007) *The Brain That Changes Itself: Stories of personal triumph from the frontiers of brain science*, Viking

Dunbar, RIM (1992) 'Neocortex Size as a Constraint on Group Size in Primates', *Journal of Human Evolution*, 22/6, 469–493, https://doi.org/10.1016/0047-2484(92)90081-J

Eaker, ED et al (2007) 'Marital Status, Marital Strain, and Risk of Coronary Heart Disease or Total Mortality: The Framingham Offspring Study', *Psychosomatic Medicine*, 69/6, 509–513, https://doi.org/10.1097/psy.0b013e3180f62357

Eisenberger, NI (2012) 'The Pain of Social Disconnection: Examining the shared neural underpinnings of physical and social pain', *Nature Reviews Neuroscience*, 13/6, 421–434, https://doi.org/10.1038/nrn3231

Eisenberger, NI et al (2011) 'Attachment Figures Activate a Safety Signal-Related Neural Region and Reduce Pain Experience', *Proceedings of the National Academy of Sciences*, 108/28, 11721–11726, https://doi.org/10.1073/pnas.1108239108

Epel, ES et al (2004) 'Accelerated Telomere Shortening in Response to Life Stress', *Proceedings of the National Academy of Sciences*, 101/49, 17312–17315, https://doi.org/10.1073/pnas.0407162101

Epel, ES et al (2009) 'Can Meditation Slow Rate of Cellular Aging? Cognitive stress, mindfulness, and telomeres', *Annals of the New York Academy of Sciences*, 1172/1, 34–53, https://doi.org/10.1111/j.1749-6632.2009.04414.x

Estruch, R et al (2018) 'Primary Prevention of Cardiovascular Disease with a Mediterranean Diet Supplemented with Extra-Virgin Olive Oil or Nuts', *New England Journal of Medicine*, 378/25, e34, https://doi.org/10.1056/nejmoa1800389

Felitti, VJ et al (1998) 'Relationship of Childhood Abuse and Household Dysfunction to Many of the Leading Causes of Death in Adults: The adverse childhood experiences (ACE) study', *American Journal of Preventive Medicine*, 14/4, 245–258, https://doi.org/10.1016/s0749-3797(98)00017-8

Fisher, HE et al (2016) 'Intense, Passionate, Romantic Love: A natural addiction? How the fields that investigate romance and substance abuse can inform each other', *Frontiers in Psychology*, 7, 687, https://doi.org/10.3389/fpsyg.2016.00687

Fontana, L, Partridge, L and Longo, VD (2010) 'Extending Healthy Life Span – From yeast to humans', *Science*, 328/5976, 321–326, https://doi.org/10.1126/science.1172539

Gallup and Rath, T (2007) *StrengthsFinder 2.0: From Gallup*, Gallup Press

Goyal, MS and Raichle, ME (2018) 'Glucose Requirements of the Developing Human Brain', *Journal of Pediatric Gastroenterology and Nutrition*, 66/3, S46–S49, https://doi.org/10.1097/MPG.0000000000001875

Hall, JA (2018) 'How Many Hours Does It Take to Make a Friend?', *Journal of Social and Personal Relationships*, 36/4, 1278–1296, https://doi.org/10.1177/0265407518761225

Harvard Second Generation Study (no date), www.adultdevelopmentstudy.org, accessed 31 December 2025

Harvie, M and Howell, T (2017) 'Potential Benefits and Harms of Intermittent Energy Restriction and

Intermittent Fasting Amongst Obese, Overweight and Normal Weight Subjects – A narrative review of human and animal evidence', *Behavioral Sciences*, 7/1, 4, https://doi.org/10.3390/bs7010004

Hebb, DO (1949) *The Organization of Behavior: A neuropsychological theory*, Wiley

Hill, N (1937) *Think and Grow Rich*, The Ralston Society

Holt-Lunstad, J, Birmingham, WA and Jones, BQ (2008) 'Is There Something Unique About Marriage? The relative impact of marital status, relationship quality, and network social support on ambulatory blood pressure and mental health', *Annals of Behavioral Medicine*, 35/2, 239–244, https://doi.org/10.1007/s12160-008-9018-y

Holt-Lunstad, J, Smith, TB and Layton, JB (2010) 'Social Relationships and Mortality Risk: A meta-analytic review', *PLoS Medicine*, 7/7, e1000316, https://doi.org/10.1371/journal.pmed.1000316

Holt-Lunstad et al (2015) 'Loneliness and Social Isolation as Risk Factors for Mortality: A meta-analytic review', Perspectivees on Psychological Science, 10/2, 227–237, https://doi.org/10.1177/1745691614568352

Hölzel, BK et al (2011) 'Mindfulness Practice Leads to Increases in Regional Brain Gray Matter Density', *Psychiatry Research: Neuroimaging*, 191/1, 36–43, https://doi.org/10.1016/j.pscychresns.2010.08.006

Jean-Berluche, D (2024) 'Creative Expression and Mental Health', *Journal of Creativity*, 34/2, 100083, https://doi.org/10.1016/j.yjoc.2024.100083

Jefferson, AL et al (2007) 'Inflammatory biomarkers are associated with total brain volume: The Framingham Heart Study', *Neurology*, 68/13, 1032–1038, https://doi.org/10.1212/01.wnl.0000257815.20548.df

Jenkinson, CE et al (2013) 'Is Volunteering a Public Health Intervention? A systematic review and meta-analysis of the health and survival of volunteers', *BMC Public Health*, 13/1, 773, https://doi.org/10.1186/1471-2458-13-773

Johnson, JB et al (2007) 'Alternate Day Calorie Restriction Improves Clinical Findings and Reduces Markers of Oxidative Stress and Inflammation in Overweight Adults with Moderate Asthma', *Free Radical Biology and Medicine*, 42/5, 665–674, https://doi.org/10.1016/j.freeradbiomed.2006.12.005

Joyce, MKP, Uchendu, S and Arnsten, AFT (2025) 'Stress and Inflammation Target Dorsolateral Prefrontal Cortex Function: Neural mechanisms underlying weakened cognitive control', *Biological Psychiatry*, 97/4, 359–371, https://doi.org/10.1016/j.biopsych.2024.06.016

Katch, V (2022) 'Healthy Pets, Healthy People', *Michigan Today*, https://michigantoday.umich.edu/2022/02/11/healthy-pets-healthy-people, accessed 1 November 2025

Kiecolt-Glaser, JK and Wilson, SJ (2017) 'Lovesick: How Couples' Relationships Influence Health', *Annual Review of Clinical Psychology*, 13, 421–443, https://doi.org/10.1146/annurev-clinpsy-032816-045111

Kiecolt-Glaser et al (2006) 'Marital Stress: Immunologic, neuroendocrine, and autonomic correlates', *Annals of Behavioral Medicine the New York Academy of Sciences*, 840/1, 656–63, https://doi.org/10.1111/j.1749-6632.1998.tb09604.x

Kolk, B van der (2014) *The Body Keeps the Score: Brain, mind, and body in the healing of trauma*, Viking

Krause, AJ et al (2017) 'The Sleep-Deprived Human Brain', *Nature Reviews Neuroscience*, 18/7, 404–418, https://doi.org/10.1038/nrn.2017.55

Lazar, SW et al (2005) 'Meditation Experience Is Associated with Increased Cortical Thickness',

NeuroReport, 16/17, 1893–1897, https://doi.org/10.1097/01.wnr.0000186598.66243.19

Lee, DH et al (2022) 'Long-Term Leisure-Time Physical Activity Intensity and All-Cause and Cause-Specific Mortality: A prospective cohort of US adults', *Circulation*, 146/7, 523–534, https://doi.org/10.1161/CIRCULATIONAHA.121.058162

Lee, H, Heller et al, (2012) 'Amygdala-prefrontal coupling underlies individual differences in emotion regulation', *NeuroImage*, 62/3, 1575–1581, https://doi.org/10.1016/j.neuroimage.2012.05.044

Lee, IM et al (2012) 'Effect of Physical Inactivity on Major Non-Communicable Diseases Worldwide: An analysis of burden of disease and life expectancy', *The Lancet*, 380/9838, 219–229, https://doi.org/10.1016/s0140-6736(12)61031-9

Lembke, A (2021) *Dopamine Nation: Finding balance in the age of indulgence*, Dutton

Lewis, T, Amini, F and Lannon, R (2000) *A General Theory of Love*, Random House

Longo, VD and Mattson, MP (2014) 'Fasting: Molecular Mechanisms and Clinical Applications', *Cell Metabolism*, 19/2, 181–192, https://doi.org/10.1016/j.cmet.2013.12.008

Longo, VD and Panda, S (2016) 'Fasting, Circadian Rhythms, and Time-Restricted Feeding in Healthy Lifespan', *Cell Metabolism*, 23/6, 1048–1059, https://doi.org/10.1016/j.cmet.2016.06.001

López-Lluch, G and Navas, P (2016) 'Calorie Restriction as an Intervention in Ageing', *Journal of Physiology*, 594/8, 2043–2060, https://doi.org/10.1113/jp270543

López-Otín, C et al (2013) 'The Hallmarks of Aging', *Cell*, 153/6, 1194–1217, https://doi.org/10.1016/j.cell.2013.05.039

López-Otín, C et al (2023) 'Hallmarks of aging: An expanding universe', *Cell*, 186/2, 243–278, https://doi.org/10.1016/j.cell.2022.11.001

Lu, Y et al (2020) 'Reprogramming to recover youthful epigenetic information and restore vision', *Nature*, 588/7836, 124–129, http://doi.org/10.1038/s41586-020-2975-4

Marsland, AL et al (2015) 'Brain Morphology Links Systemic Inflammation to Cognitive Function in Midlife Adults', *Brain, Behavior, and Immunity*, 48, 195–204, https://doi.org/10.1016/j.bbi.2015.03.015

Master, SL et al (2009) 'A Picture's Worth: Partner photographs reduce experimentally induced pain',

Psychological Science, 20/11, 1316–1318, https://doi.org/10.1111/j.1467-9280.2009.02444.x

Mattison, JA et al (2017) 'Caloric Restriction Improves Health and Survival of Rhesus Monkeys', *Nature Communications*, 8, 14063, https://doi.org/10.1038/ncomms14063

Mattson, MP et al (2018) 'Intermittent Metabolic Switching, Neuroplasticity and Brain Health', *Nature Reviews Neuroscience*, 19/2, 81–94, https://doi.org/10.1038/nrn.2017.156

Mattson, MP, Longo VD and Harvie M (2017) 'Impact of Intermittent Fasting on Health and Disease Processes', *Ageing Research Reviews*, 39, 46–58, https://doi.org/10.1016/j.arr.2016.10.005

McGaugh, JL (2004) 'The Amygdala Modulates the Consolidation of Memories of Emotionally Arousing Experiences', *Annual Review of Neuroscience*, 27, 1–28, https://doi.org/10.1146/annurev.neuro.27.070203.144157

Merzenich, M (2013) *Soft-Wired: How the new science of brain plasticity can change your life*, Parnassus Publishing

Merzenich, M, Van Vleet, TM and Nahum, M (2014) 'Brain Plasticity-Based Therapeutics', *Frontiers in*

Human Neuroscience, 8, 385, https://doi.org/10.3389/fnhum.2014.00385

Miller, AH (2009) 'Mechanisms of Cytokine-Induced Behavioral Changes: Psychoneuroimmunology at the translational interface', *Brain, Behavior, and Immunity*, 23/2, 149–158, https://doi.org/10.1016/j.bbi.2008.08.006

Mizushima, N et al (2008) 'Autophagy Fights Disease Through Cellular Self-Digestion', *Nature*, 451/7182, 1069–1075, https://doi.org/10.1038/nature06639

Monteiro, CA et al (2019) 'Ultra-Processed Foods: What they are and how to identify them', *Public Health Nutrition*, 22/5, 936–941, https://doi.org/10.1017/s1368980018003762

Myers, P and Briggs Myers, I (1995) *Gifts Differing: Understanding personality type*, John Murray Business

Neff, KD (2003) 'Self-Compassion: An alternative conceptualization of a healthy attitude toward oneself', *Self and Identity*, 2/2, 85–101, http://dx.doi.org/10.1080/15298860309032

Ohsumi, Y (2014) 'Historical Landmarks of Autophagy Research', *Cell Research*, 24/1, 9–23, https://doi.org/10.1038/cr.2013.169

Pariante, CM (2017) 'Why Are Depressed Patients Inflamed? A reflection on 20 years of research on depression, glucocorticoid resistance and inflammation', *European Neuropsychopharmacology*, 27/6, 554–559, https://doi.org/10.1016/j.euroneuro.2017.04.001

Pavlov, IP (1927) *Conditioned Reflexes: An investigation of the physiological activity of the cerebral cortex*, Oxford University Press

Pennebaker, JW (1997) 'Writing About Emotional Experiences as a Therapeutic Process', *Psychological Science*, 8/3, 162–166, https://doi.org/10.1111/j.1467-9280.1997.tb00403.x

Pert, CB (1997) *Molecules of Emotion: The science behind mind-body medicine*, Scribner

Pert, CB et al (1985) 'Neuropeptides and Their Receptors: A psychosomatic network', *Journal of Immunology*, 135/2, 820–826, https://doi.org/10.4049/jimmunol.135.2.820

Primack, BA et al (2017) 'Social Media Use and Perceived Social Isolation Among Young Adults in the US', *American Journal of Preventive Medicine*, 53/1, 1–8, https://doi.org/10.1016/j.amepre.2017.01.010

Raison, CL and Miller, AH (2013) 'Malaise, Melancholia and Madness: The evolutionary legacy of an inflammatory bias', *Brain, Behaviour, and Immunity*, 31, 1–8, https://doi.org/10.1016/j.bbi.2013.04.009

Rajman, L, Chwalek, K and Sinclair, DA (2018) 'Therapeutic Potential of NAD-Boosting Molecules: The *in vivo* evidence', *Cell Metabolism*, 27/3, 529–547, https://doi.org/10.1016/j.cmet.2018.02.011

Rakel, D et al (2011) 'Perception of Empathy in the Therapeutic Encounter: Effects on the common cold', *Patient Education and Counseling*, 85/3, 390–397, https://doi.org/10.1016/j.pec.2011.01.009

Ratey, JJ (2008) *Spark: The revolutionary new science of exercise and the brain*, Little, Brown and Company

Reis, HT and Shaver, P (1988) 'Intimacy as an Interpersonal Process', in S Duck et al (eds) *Handbook of Personal Relationships: Theory, research and interventions*, Wiley & Sons, 367–389

Rico-Campà, A et al (2019) 'Association Between Consumption of Ultra-Processed Foods and All Cause Mortality: SUN prospective cohort study', *British Medical Journal*, 365, l1949, https://doi.org/10.1136/bmj.l1949

Riso, DR and Hudson, R (1999) *The Wisdom of the Enneagram: The complete guide to psychological and spiritual growth for the nine personality types*, Bantam

Robes, TF et al (2014) 'Marital Quality and Health: A meta-analytic review', *Psychological Bulletin*, 140/1, 140–187, https://doi.org/10.1037/a0031859

Rosen, DS et al (2024) 'Creative Flow as Optimized Processing: Evidence from brain oscillations during jazz improvisations by expert and non-expert musicians', *Neuropsychologia*, 196, 108824, https://doi.org/10.1016/j.neuropsychologia.2024.108824

Rubinsztein, DC, Mariño, G and Kroemer, G (2011) 'Autophagy and Aging', *Cell*, 146/5, 682–695, https://doi.org/10.1016/j.cell.2011.07.030

Ruiz-González, D et al (2021) 'Effects of physical exercise on plasma brain-derived neurotrophic factor in neurodegenerative disorders: A systematic review and meta-analysis of randomized controlled trials', *Neuroscience & Biobehavioural Reviews*, 128, 394–405, https://doi.org/10.1016/j.neubiorev.2021.05.025

Rutter, M (2012) 'Resilience as a Dynamic Concept', *Development and Psychopathology*, 24/2, 335–344, https://doi.org/10.1017/s0954579412000028

Saliev, T and Singh, PB (2025) 'Targeting Senescence: A review of senolytics and senomorphics in anti-aging interventions'. *Biomolecules*, 15/6, 860. https://doi.org/10.3390/biom15060860

Sapolsky, RM (2004) *Why Zebras Don't Get Ulcers: The acclaimed guide to stress, stress-related diseases, and coping*, 3rd ed, Henry Holt and Company

Sapolsky, RM (2017) *Behave: The biology of humans at our best and worst*, Penguin Press

Seltzer, LJ, Ziegler, TE and Pollak, SD (2010) 'Social Vocalizations Can Release Oxytocin in Humans', *Proceedings of the Royal Society B*, 277/1694, 2661–2666, https://doi.org/10.1098/rspb.2010.0567

Shakya, HB and Christakis, NA (2017) 'Association of Facebook Use with Compromised Well-Being: A longitudinal study', *American Journal of Epidemiology*, 185/3, 203–211, https://doi.org/10.1093/aje/kww189

Sinclair, DA and LaPlante, MD (2019) *Lifespan: Why We Age – And why we don't have to*, Atria Books

Sommerlad, A et al (2023) 'Social Participation and Risk of Developing Dementia', *Nature Aging*, 3, 532–545, https://doi.org/10.1038/s43587-023-00387-0

Šrámek, P et al (2000) 'Human Physiological Responses to Immersion into Water of Different Temperatures', *European Journal of Applied Physiology*, 81/5, 436–442, https://doi.org/10.1007/s004210050065

Srour, B et al (2019) 'Ultra-Processed Food Intake and Risk of Cardiovascular Disease: Prospective cohort study (NutriNet-Santé)', *British Medical Journal*, 365, l1451, https://doi.org/10.1136/bmj.l1451

Stellar, JE et al (2015) 'Positive Affect and Markers of Inflammation: Discrete positive emotions predict lower levels of inflammatory cytokines', *Emotion*, 15/2, 129–133, https://doi.org/10.1037/emo0000033

Stephens, GJ, Silbert, LJ and Hasson, U (2010) 'Speaker–Listener Neural Coupling Underlies Successful Communication', *Proceedings of the National Academy of Sciences*, 107/32, 14425–14430, https://doi.org/10.1073/pnas.1008662107

Tang, YY et al (2007) 'Short-Term Meditation Training Improves Attention and Self-Regulation', *Proceedings of the National Academy of Sciences*, 104/43, 17152–17156, https://doi.org/10.1073/pnas.0707678104

Waldinger, R and Shulz, M (2023) *The Good Life: Lessons from the World's Longest Study on Happiness*, Simon & Schuster

Weisman, O et al (2014) 'Early Stage Romantic Love Is Associated with Reduced Daily Cortisol Production', *Adaptive Human Behavior and Physiology*, 1/1, 41–53, https://doi.org/10.1007/s40750-014-0007-z

WHO (2025a) 'Loneliness and Isolation – The hidden threat to global health we can no longer ignore' (World Health Organization Commission on Social

Connection, Geneva), www.who.int/news-room/commentaries/detail/loneliness-and-isolation-the-hidden-threat-to-global-health-we-can-no-longer-ignore, accessed 10 January 2026

WHO (2025b) 'From Loneliness to Social Connection' (World Health Organization Commission on Social Connection, Geneva), www.who.int/publications/i/item/978240112360, accessed 19 January 2026

Willcox, BJ, Willcox, DC and Suzuki, M (2007) *The Okinawa Program: How the world's longest-lived people achieve everlasting health and how you can too*, National Geographic Society

Woollett, K and Maguire, EA (2011) 'Acquiring "the Knowledge" of London's Layout Drives Structural Brain Changes', *Current Biology*, 21/24, 2109–2114, https://doi.org/10.1016/j.cub.2011.11.018

Further Reading

Adams, KM et al (2006) 'Status of Nutrition Education in Medical Schools: A cross-sectional study', *The American Journal of Clinical Nutrition*, 83/4, 941S–944S, https://doi.org/10.1093/ajcn/83.4.941s

American College of Lifestyle Medicine, www.lifestylemedicine.org, accessed 30 September 2025

Areta, JL et al (2013) 'Timing and Distribution of Protein Ingestion During Prolonged Recovery from Resistance Exercise Alters Myofibrillar Protein Synthesis', *Journal of Physiology*, 591/9, 2319–2331, https://doi.org/10.1113/jphysiol.2012.244897

Bably, Z et al (2025) 'Mindfulness-Based Interventions and Neuroplasticity: A review of network connectivity in healthy and clinical samples', *Mindfulness*, 16/4, 783–796, https://doi.org/10.1007/s12671-025-02549-0

Blackburn, EH, Epel, ES and Lin J (2015) 'Human Telomere Biology: A contributory and interactive factor in aging, cardiovascular disease risks, and protection', *Science*, 350/6265, 1193–1198, https://doi.org/10.1126/science.aab3389

Blue Zones, www.bluezones.com, accessed 30 September 2025

Braverman, ER (2004) *The Edge Effect: Achieve total health and longevity with the balanced brain advantage*, Sterling Publishing

Brown, B (2010) *The Gifts of Imperfection*, Hazelden Publishing

Brown, LL, Acevedo, B and Fisher, HE (2013) 'Neural Correlates of Four Broad Temperament Dimensions: Testing predictions for a novel construct of personality', *PLoS One*, 8/11, e78734, https://doi.org/10.1371/journal.pone.0078734

Cantó, C and Auwerx, J (2009) 'PGC-1α, SIRT1 and AMPK, an Energy Sensing Network That Controls Energy Expenditure', *Current Opinion in Lipidology*, 20/2, 98–105, https://doi.org/10.1097/mol.0b013e328328d0a4

Cantó, C, Menzies, KJ and Auwerx J (2013) 'NAD+ Metabolism and the Control of Energy Homeostasis: A balancing act between mitochondria and the nucleus', *Cell Metabolism*, 22/1, 31–53, https://doi.org/10.1016/j.cmet.2015.05.023

Crowley, J, Ball, L and Hiddink, GJ (2019) 'Nutrition Education in Medical Schools: A systematic review', *The Lancet Planetary Health*, 3/9, E379–E389, https://doi.org/10.1016/s2542-5196(19)30171-8

Csikszentmihalyi, M (1990) *Flow: The psychology of optimal experience*, Harper & Row

Duckworth, A (2016) *Grit: The power of passion and perseverance*, Scribner

Franceschi, C et al (2018) 'Inflammaging: A new immune-metabolic viewpoint for age-related diseases', *Nature Reviews Endocrinology*, 14/10, 576–590, https://doi.org/10.1038/s41574-018-0059-4

Freeman, AM et al (2017) 'Trending Cardiovascular Nutrition Controversies', *Journal of the American College of Cardiology*, 69/9, 1172–1187, https://doi.org/10.1016/j.jacc.2016.10.086

Gilbert, E (2015) *Big Magic: Creative living beyond fear*, Riverhead Books

Goodyear, VA et al (2021) 'The effect of social media interventions on physical activity and dietary behaviours in young people and adults: A systematic review', *International Journal of Behavioral Nutrition and Physical Activity*, 18, 72, https://doi.org/10.1186/s12966-021-01138-3

Harvard Health Publishing, www.health.harvard.edu, accessed 30 September 2025

Harvie, MN et al (2011) 'The Effects of Intermittent or Continuous Energy Restriction on Weight Loss and Metabolic Disease Risk Markers: A randomized trial in young overweight women', *International Journal of Obesity*, 35/5, 714–727, https://doi.org/10.1038/ijo.2010.171

Institute for Functional Medicine, www.ifm.org, accessed 30 September 2025

Jiménez-Cortegana, C et al (2021) 'Nutrients and Dietary Approaches in Patients with Type 2 Diabetes Mellitus and Cardiovascular Disease: A Narrative Review' *Nutrients*, 13/11, 4150, https://doi.org/10.3390/nu13114150

Kiecolt-Glaser, JK, Gouin, JP and Hantsoo, L (2010) 'Close Relationships, Inflammation, and Health', *Neuroscience and Biobehavioral Reviews*, 35/1, 33–38, https://doi.org/10.1016/j.neubiorev.2009.09.003

Kiecolt-Glaser, JK et al (2005) 'Hostile Marital Interactions, Proinflammatory Cytokine Production, and Wound Healing', *Archives of General Psychiatry*, 62/12, 1377–1384, https://doi.org/10.1001/archpsyc.62.12.1377

Lieberman, MD (2013) *Social: Why our brains are wired to connect*, Crown Publishers

Luchetti, M et al (2024) 'A Meta-Analysis of Loneliness and Risk of Dementia Using Longitudinal Data from >600,000 Individuals', *Nature Mental Health*, 2/11, 1350–1361, https://doi.org/10.1038/s44220-024-00328-9

Mayo Clinic, www.mayoclinic.org/healthy-lifestyle, accessed 30 September 2025

Mednick, S (2006) *Take a Nap! Change your life*, Workman Publishing

Moore, DR et al (2009) 'Ingested Protein Dose Response of Muscle and Albumin Protein Synthesis After Resistance Exercise in Young Men', *American Journal of Clinical* Nutrition, 89/1, 161–168, https://doi.org/10.3945/ajcn.2008.26401

Neff, KD (2011) *Self-Compassion: The proven power of being kind to yourself*, William Morrow

Paddon-Jones, D et al (2008) 'Role of Dietary Protein in the Sarcopenia of Aging', *American Journal of Clinical Nutrition*, 87/5, 1562S–1566S, https://doi.org/10.1093/ajcn/87.5.1562s

Patterson, RE et al (2015) 'Intermittent Fasting and Human Metabolic Health', *Journal of the Academy of Nutrition and Dietetics*, 115/8, 1203–1212, https://doi.org/10.1016/j.jand.2015.02.018

Pedersen, BK and Saltin, B (2015) 'Exercise as Medicine – Evidence for prescribing exercise as therapy in 26 different chronic diseases', *Scandinavian Journal of Medicine and Science in Sports*, 25/S3, 1–72, https://doi.org/10.1111/sms.12581

Phillips, SM and Van Loon, LJ (2011) 'Dietary Protein for Athletes: From requirements to optimum adaptation', *Journal of Sports Sciences*, 29/S1, S29–S38, https://doi.org/10.1080/02640414.2011.619204

Roenneberg, T (2012) *Internal Time: Chronotypes, social jet lag, and why you're so tired*, Harvard University Press

Schachner, DA, Shaver, PR and Mikulincer, M (2005) 'Patterns of Nonverbal Behavior and Sensitivity in the Context of Attachment Relations', *Journal of Nonverbal Behavior*, 29/3, 141–169, http://dx.doi.org/10.1007/s10919-005-4847-x

Seshadri, S et al (2002) 'Plasma Homocysteine as a Risk Factor for Dementia and Alzheimer's Disease', *New England Journal of Medicine*, 346/7, 476–483, https://doi.org/10.1056/nejmoa011613

Sinek, S (2009) *Start With Why: How great leaders inspire everyone to take action*, Portfolio

Tinsley, GM and La Bounty, PM (2015) 'Effects of Intermittent Fasting on Body Composition and

Clinical Health Markers in Humans', *Nutrition Reviews*, 73/10, 661–74, https://doi.org/10.1093/nutrit/nuv041

Walker, KA et al (2017) 'Midlife Systemic Inflammatory Markers Are Associated with Late-Life Brain Volume: The ARIC study', *Neurology*, 89/22, 2262–2270, https://doi.org/10.1212/wnl.0000000000004688

Walker, M (2017) *Why We Sleep: Unlocking the power of sleep and dreams*, Simon & Schuster

Acknowledgements

This book has been years in the making – a distillation of personal transformation, clinical experience and hard-won insights. Writing it has been an act of healing, and my hope is that it serves you in your own journey.

Thanks to every patient who has shown me their private depths and hopes; you have been my greatest teachers. I have found resilience within your suffering. I have seen you make miracles in your healing. You have each permanently impressed my soul. Everyone I have met along the way – from prisons and tension-filled boardrooms to the sacred space of the consulting room or operating theatre – has handed me a lesson in what it means to be human, though admittedly not always when I was fully aware.

I owe the scientific foundation of the hope I offer in these pages to the work of countless researchers, and I hold them all in my highest regard. Your commitment to truth telling anchors the dreams we have of change.

To my family and friends, who watched me give up everything I'd thought I wanted for a then undefined dream: thank you for putting up with my restless soul. You understood on some level, before I even did, that sometimes we must lose ourselves entirely to find what we are truly meant for.

I will be forever grateful to my parents, who live forever within me. They believed in me when I had no faith in myself, and their faith has carried me through the wilderness of becoming. Also to my beloved siblings, nephews and nieces in Spain; even though you are far away, your love supports me. You are the roots that keep me grounded, reminding me where I come from and who I am, beneath any title and achievement.

I am so lucky that my family has grown to include more than just blood and DNA. I have a wonderful wider family circle – the Carrs, Sacks and many more. Thank you for loving me and nurturing me every day.

To my dearest rock, SF: I am forever indebted to you for your unwavering support and the light you bring to my world.

This book would never have come to life without three souls who altered everything:

JPG, my guru, my very own Peter Pan and unlimited love giver, who taught me that life is not about enduring but about finding the adventure. You took up my cause when I had lost faith in myself; you taught me that play and purpose can dance together in the most beautiful ways.

PMC, who made me whole, loved and reminded me of my own worth. Your departure left an unimaginable hole, and nothing seems to be able to fill it. You are always present in all that I do. The love you left spreads everywhere, and the pain of your departure is compensated by the gift of having known someone like you.

JB, who, without even trying or ever speaking, opened something inside of me. Although we took separate roads, I will forever be in debt to you for the oceans you awoke.

Finally, my thanks go to you, dear reader. For picking up this book and being courageous enough to peer into your own life and have faith that change is achievable. The knowledge that someone out there might be brave enough to embark on the journey of transformation has made every challenge I have faced in life worthwhile. Let these pages be your trusted friend as you gently step higher on the path to living fully, authentically, and beautifully becoming you.

The Author

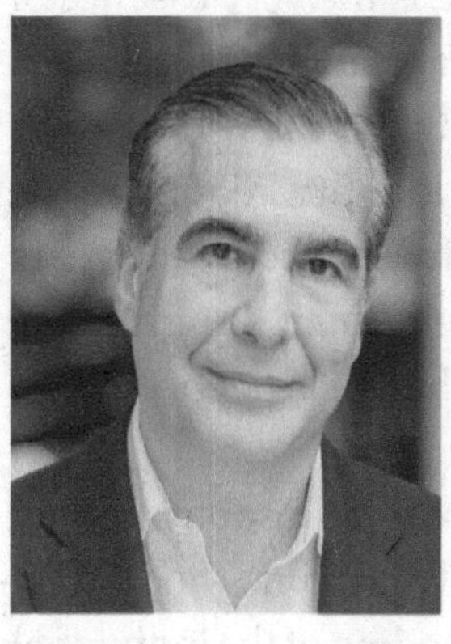

Dr J Crespo is a GP working in private practice and at the NHS Chelsea and Westminster Hospital's A&E department. He has also been a clinical teacher and examiner for Imperial College, London. His career has spanned many countries, job roles and situations, which represents the depth of transformation he illustrates in this book.

Even though he was always passionate about healing and transforming the world, his dream of becoming a doctor was derailed by personal circumstances, leading him first to become a lawyer. A few years after, he decided to leave his native Spain – never to return – and went on to further train in finance. He undertook assignments around the globe as a consultant for

Towers Perrin, a director for Standard & Poor's and also running the European business as general manager of AM Best in London.

An epiphany encouraged him to risk everything and take the leap into medicine, starting again almost from scratch. The determination with which he commanded his previous metamorphoses enabled him once more to progress rapidly in his new field.

His journey, from a Spanish law student to a British financial executive then a doctor, is the very essence of neuroplasticity and the human capacity for reinvention about which he writes in this book. Each transition was a stripping down of an old identity, requiring the learning of new skills and humility shaped by the years it would take to understand the human struggles we confront when we decide that change is needed.

Dr J Crespo maintains his medical philosophy, rooted in combining effective biological and mind–body treatments with a humanistic understanding of the individual. This comes from understanding that healing addresses not only symptoms but the whole person – biology, psychology, emotions, relationships and life circumstances. His own journey across continents, languages, professions and worlds echoes the principles he imparts: that deep transformation is always possible when one gains a grounded knowledge of, and commitment to, life.

🌐 www.drjcrespo.com

www.ingramcontent.com/pod-product-compliance
Lightning Source LLC
LaVergne TN
LVHW030919080826
845145LV00013B/2969

* 9 7 8 1 7 8 1 3 3 9 6 1 9 *